Praise for LADIES OF THE KASBAH

'Mullins' chief aim is to put the case for legalised brothels, And to complain - with perfect justice - that whereas it was the girls who suffered legal persecution their clients...leading figures in the political, commercial, judicial and ecclesiastical life...escaped unscathed... Who among our legislators will have the courage to answer these calls of reason, and do something about it?'

Financial Times

It deserves to sell because it is a record of social history. The Kasbah flourished for over a decade when the country - and huge numbers of politicians, legal people, and other opinion shapers who used the sumptuously sleazy brothel for any amount of deviant sex - was convulsed in hysterics about the exact time of ensoulment of a foetus, abortion and divorce...this book confirms the belief that the *Pretty Woman* and *Klute* versions of their [prostitutes'] lives are in the land of Cinderella and other fairy tales'

Irish Times

'A riveting story...taking the lid of yet another sleazy, secretive aspect of Irish life'

Sunday Independent

'Now, for the first time, a new book lifts the lid off the sordid and shocking world behind the doors of this basement bordello'

Star

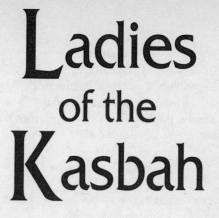

Ladies
of the
Kasbah

Dave Mullins

WARNER BOOKS

A *Warner* Book

First published in Great Britain in 1995 by
Little, Brown and Company
This edition published in 1996 by Warner Books
Reprinted 1997

Copyright © Dave Mullins 1995

The moral right of the author has been asserted.

A CIP catalogue record for this book is available
from the British Library.

ISBN 0 7515 1642 2

Printed and bound in Great Britain by
Clays Ltd, St Ives plc

Warner Books
A Division of
Little, Brown and Company (UK)
Brettenham House
Lancaster Place
London WC2E 7EN

To: Mary my wife,
for your love with understanding;

our children,
for your love without it;

and, of course, the Ladies of the Kasbah,
for a journey into the unknown

Acknowledgements

Many who deserve my gratitude must, for their own good reasons, go unacknowledged in print: this sentiment does little to meet their goodness to me and value to this book.

There is a woman called Kate whose words of skill and care and support were of immense importance to me during my trials of little self-belief. The *Sunday World* newspaper and its staff provided invaluable time and facilities, particularly in the research area. My colleague, Séan Boyne, is owed special thanks for being both officer and gentleman in the collaborative process of the book and afterwards. I am in the debt of other friends and colleagues for their tolerance and feedback.

Tom Cooney of the Law Faculty in University College, Dublin, provided me with vital insights into the dynamics of vice-related law with a willingness to assist which was in itself an education. My many friends in the legal profession also applied themselves with remarkable mastery and enthusiasm.

I must also acknowledge those whom I approached for help with this book but who felt unable to give it. I have done my best to temper my disappointment with understanding. I hope I have succeeded.

Contents

Prologue

The characters in this book are all real – although in many instances their identities have been concealed for a variety of reasons. The Kasbah women named herein as Linda Lavelle, Vikki O'Toole, Lis O'Brien, Charlene Robertson and Pia Masterson, are, for instance, aliases attributed to the women by the author.

Names such as Marion Murphy, Margaret Healy and Liz Brophy and others are bona fide as are all names used in historical, legal and other contextual extracts including those of all the police officers. The many and varied clients to the bordello bear the same eccentric titles bestowed on them by their prostitute women.

Any similarity between the aliased characters in this book and persons living and not connected with it defies the author's painstaking attempts to avoid such a happening and is purely coincidental.

Introduction

A Woman Cheated

This is the story of a small group of Irish women and the men they serve.

It is an odyssey into a hidden modern Ireland of sex and sadomasochism in the 1980s and 1990s – the story of a place called the Kasbah, Ireland's most infamous brothel, scene of The Politician In The Massage Parlour Scandal which rocked the nation back in late 1991.

It is, I believe, a story of national significance for Ireland.

Until its closure in October of the same year the Kasbah was home to the secret fantasies of men: powerful men and ordinary men, rich men and poor men.

It was never just paid sex that made the Kasbah what it was for over a decade. The bulk of the 120 or so men who passed through the doors of this basement brothel at 60B Mountjoy Square West in the heart of Dublin city every single week sipped from a trough of sexual deviance so extreme as to be at first incredible.

The customers' clandestine visits to the Kasbah seldom if ever were made for the purpose of straight sex, preferring as they did the often atrocious à la carte versions of perversion, kink and fantasy and other forms of deviance. It is this predilection to perversity which is at once the saddest, funniest and most disturbing facet of this book: these covert visits down the basement steps of a run-down Georgian building in a run-down part of Dublin were made by men wanting to live out the most lurid fantasies for which large sums of cash were gratefully paid.

I have spent three years investigating the goings-on at the Kasbah and the prostitutes who work there under the watchful tutelage of their Madam, Linda Lavelle [not her real name], Ireland's undisputed First Lady of Vice.

My wildest imaginings could not have prepared me for what I would discover in countless hours of interviews with Linda and many other prostitutes. Time and time again, household names were trundled out: politicians, leading Church figures, businessmen, stalwarts of the legal profession.

The Kasbah's final closure was just as bizarre and unbelievable as anything that went on there during the ten torrid years of its existence, involving as it did the most unlikely figure of former Post Office clerk John Keegan who had become known without affection by the girls as 'Little John'. Keegan managed to spend an incredible £12,000 in just eight months on one of the Kasbah girls – Margaret 'Poppy' Healy. When the money ran out, so did Poppy, and Little John's mind turned from boyish sexual infatuation to revenge, conducting as he did a one-man hate campaign against the Kasbah and its inhabitants with ruthless efficiency. It was to result in the biggest anti-vice police surveillance operation in the history of the State and lead to a three-day criminal trial in 1993.

It was as I sat with a betrayed Linda Lavelle outside the large wooden doors of Circuit Criminal Court Number 15 in the Four Courts – the epicentre of the Irish legal system – that between us the idea for this book was conceived. 'Why,' she asked, 'are we always the fucking underdogs?'

This was never intended as a definitive document on prostitution; nor as an ideological stand on behalf of the vice girls. To do that, I felt, would be to subsume the individuality of the Kasbah women.

Neither is this a book that is going to name names – on either side of the sexual market place. Rightly or wrongly, I have decided that identifying anyone whose name is not already part of the public domain serves no real purpose and would also serve to hurt the women who gave so much to me as I researched this book and who asked for nothing in return other than that their identities be kept secret.

This is then, quite simply, the story of Linda Lavelle and the girls who, for better or for worse, in sickness and in health, drunk or strung-out, worked at the Kasbah. It is a testimony, too, to the men – the clients – and their sexual zealousness: sometimes perverse, sometimes spectacular, sometimes hilarious, sometimes pathetic and always shocking. It is also an attempt to understand what goes on in the conscious and subconscious minds of such men, many of whom hold supremely high office in Ireland today.

In that respect it is a deeply disturbing account of private Irish lives.

If this is an outrageous book it is so only because it is a book of outrageous behaviour. Above all, it is a story that deserves to be told. There is a sense of enormous privilege within me in its telling. I hope I have remained faithful to Linda Lavelle, her beloved Kasbah and the girls who worked there, with their disarming candour and scorn, their compassion, their humanity and, perhaps above all, their exquisitely merciless sense of humour.

Dave Mullins
Dublin, 1994

Chapter One

'Girls, It's A Raid!'

To a casual observer the incident might have looked more like a scene from an old Pink Panther movie with Peter Sellers as Inspector Clouseau than the deadly serious and professional police operation that it was. Ten burly officers led by Detective Inspector Michael Duggan pulled up outside the run-down Georgian building in north inner-city Dublin. Detectives Kevin Fields and Gus Keane, the main investigating officers, were there, as were police specialists from the photographic and mapping sections of police headquarters, laden with cases of technical paraphernalia. Five other officers of varying ranks made up the numbers.

Inspector Duggan and Detective Fields descended the basement steps of the two-storey premises brandishing a search warrant while the rest of the force remained above on the litter swept footpath in this part of Dublin city which can seem so empty and undernourished. The main entrance door was ajar: the two cops entered a dimly lit hallway, where, as written police evidence would later quirkily recall, 'We were met by a second door'. Inspector Duggan knocked firmly.

Silence.

A female voice from within the locked recesses of the bordello known as Laura's Studio eventually rasped out, 'We're busy, come back in half an hour!' The two spurned policemen looked at each other before deciding to rejoin the posse on the roadside, the warrant issued by District Court Judge Brian Kirby still unserved.

They considered their options.

The police chief and his bemused crew had little real cause for concern. It was 1.20pm on a muggy and overcast Wednesday afternoon, 4 September 1991. If needs be, the search could wait, as most of the officers felt that the case against Marion Murphy of brothel-keeping was already virtually in the can thanks to a surveillance operation which spanned 5 July to 20 August in which more than 123 men had been video-taped entering and leaving Laura's Studio at 24 Belvedere Place and a similar basement premises at Number 60B in nearby Mountjoy Square West – the infamous Kasbah. Thirteen of the quaintly named clients who were subsequently filmed gave signed depositions to the lower courts to the effect that they had partaken of various forms of sexual services in exchange for money at either Laura's or the Kasbah on the dates on which they had been covertly filmed by the police.

The securely parcelled cassette tapes containing film of the majority of the clients sighted were handed over to Detective Dominic Hutchin at police headquarters in Harcourt Square at noon on Monday 12 August: it was at that precise moment, as the midday bells of the Angelus pealed out over the old grey city of Dublin, that the die was cast, both for Marion Murphy, and for an era unparalleled in Irish prostitution that she, however unwittingly, and the girls who worked for her, were responsible for bringing about.

Inspector Duggan and his team hadn't long to wait as they stood on the pavement outside 24 Belvedere Place. After a few minutes, Marion and her then good friend and manageress Margaret 'Poppy' Healy arrived at Laura's in Poppy's 1990 black Renault 19 en route from the Kasbah, oblivious to the presence of ten frustrated officers of the State standing outside their brothel. Marion Murphy coolly got out of the car, walked over to the assemblage of uniformed officers and told them that she had the keys to the locked inside door and would gladly open it. She went with officers Duggan and Fields back down the concrete steps. Without warning, she jumped the final four steps, ran into the hall and banged a window with both her fists, yelling, 'Girls, it's a raid. It's the police. Don't open up.' Two detectives who had joined them forced the door open as Detective Fields stood between Ms Murphy and the window. Three girls were interviewed inside. Handbags were searched and condoms found ('They're for personal use, officer'.)

There were no real surprises. A notebook with a limp £10 note hanging out of it and containing the words 'S and Massage' beside a string of men's names was explained by Ms Murphy as 'Shower and Massage' as she protested with the police saying that the book was personal, containing such details as her parents' address.

It was all grist-to-the-mill evidential stuff needed to secure a conviction for the forthcoming trial which would witness Marion Murphy continue her protestations of innocence. She never once contested the claims that the Kasbah was being operated as a brothel. Her defence was that she had *no knowledge* of that fact, asserting as she did that the basement of 60B Mountjoy Square West was being run by her through her manageresses, Linda Lavelle and Poppy Healy, as a bona fide health and fitness studio.

On 6 September, less than forty-eight hours after the raid on 24 Belvedere Place, Marion Murphy arrived at the busy inner-city Fitzgibbon Street police station where she was received by Detective Sergeant Timothy Daly and Detective Kevin Fields. She had made the appointment herself after earlier declining to make a statement to the police about their investigations into an alleged brothel. She sat impassively on one side of a rectangular and well-worn table as the two police

officers prepared themselves in the small interview room. Daly
would ask the questions. Fields would record and transcribe.

Daly: What do you work at?
Murphy: A masseuse.
D: Where do you work from?
M: 24, Belvedere Place, in the basement.
D: How many people, girls, do you employ?
M: Four girls there.
D: Can you name them?
M: [She offers four female Christian names and one surname]
D: How much do you pay these girls a week?
M: They're on commission.
D: How does the commission work?
M: £5 per customer.
D: Are they permanent staff?
M: Yes.
D: How many massage rooms have you there?
M: Three and a waiting room.
D: On 4/9/91 we met you outside the door of 24. I asked you
did you have keys. I asked if you'd let us in. You said yes.
Why didn't you let us in?
M: I didn't have keys.
D: Why didn't ya [*sic*] ask the girls to let us in?
M: Not really [*sic*].
D: Why did you shout to the girls 'Girls, it's a raid, it's the
police'?
M: I can't remember shouting that.
D: Did you know who we were?
M: I thought you were the carpet layers. I didn't recognise you,
(pointing to Daly) until the last minute.
D: Why is there steel gates erected between the reception
room and the massage rooms?
M: To curtail people wrecking the place!
D: Why did you say to me 'If you came in a few days time

you'll get no further than the gate'?

M: I don't recall saying that.

D: Did you ever have TVs [television sets] in the room?

M: We used to do keep fit classes.

D: Is there sex been [*sic*] offered to any of the clients at 24 Belvedere Place?

M: Oh Jesus! No.

D: How do you account for the book Detective Fields is showing you, the wire bound notebook with entries reading 'S and Massage £15'?

M: That's shower and massage.

D: Are you in complete charge of the basement at 24 Belvedere Place?

M: Yes.

D: Have you any connections with 60B Mountjoy Square?

M: Yes, I rent and run a Health Studio called the Kasbah there.

D: Who manages that for you?

M: I am the overseer [pointing to herself].

D: How many girls work there for you?

M: Basically four.

D: Who are they?

M: [Ms Murphy gives four female Christian names and three surnames]

D: How much do you pay for renting 60B?

M: £60.

D: Who have you rented these premises from?

M: B. O'Gara*, West of Ireland.

D: Do you have a lease?

M: Yes, but in the name Vicki Collins.†

D: Why do you have the lease in a false name?

M: For no particular reason.

---

*The lease dated 20 November 1982, was, in fact, signed by Noel O'Gara of Ballinahown Court, Athlone, County Westmeath.

†The signature 'Vickie Collins' was written by Marion Murphy.

D: Is there sex offered to clients or callers?

M: Oh! No.

D: Do you yourself do massages at these premises?

M: I have at both places.

D: We have statements from callers to 60B Mountjoy Square stating that they (men) had been offered and partook and paid for sexual favours from the staff there. Can you account for this?

M: There is no sexual favours or anything like that been [*sic*] offered.

D: We have a statement from one man who says he paid for a . . . sexual favours from yourself at 60B Mountjoy Square.

M: Definitely not.

D: How long is Mountjoy Square in operation?

M: Eight and a half years.

D: And 24 Belvedere Place?

M: Five years.

D: Are you involved in any other health studio?

M: No.

D: How is the money collected if you are based at 24 Belvedere Place?

M: Margaret Healy brings it sometimes. Otherwise I get it myself.

D: Are you a qualified masseuse?

M: Yes. These are my qualifications.

D: The rubbish bags that were taken at number 24. Can you account for anything in them or found in them, i.e. an empty condom box?

M: No.

D: Is that all ya [*sic*] wish to say?

M: Yes.

D: Do you wish to sign these notes?

M: Yes.

D: Are they correct?

M: Yes.

What Inspector Duggan and his investigators couldn't have known, as they continued their attempts to gain access to the premises in Belvedere Place, is how different, how bizarre, their evidence would have been if they had timed their raid three days earlier and had started their descent down the iron steps of the Kasbah instead of Laura's. For on that prior Sunday, Linda Lavelle and her girls were conducting one of their regular 'Madhatters' Nights' in which this most exquisitely sinful arena was turned into a sanctuary for collective sexual fantasy.

As I sat in the press box during Marion Murphy's trial in the Dublin Circuit Criminal Court in February 1993 I couldn't help imagining the horror and disbelief on the faces of the jury of eight women and four men at such an encounter being recalled in evidence by a stony faced police officer to Judge Gerard Buchanan in the hushed giant courtroom.

'Upon entering the premises, Your Honour, I observed seven adult males in a state of complete undress suspended from the ceiling by a metal loop. They had chains tied to their wrists which tailed around their private parts. The men appeared to be in a state of sexual arousal, Your Honour. Some of them were moaning and others were shouting obscenities.'

The evidence might very well have been completed thus, 'On a bed on the floor and directly in front of aforementioned males, Your Honour, I observed two adult females, also in a state of complete undress, who were clutched together, one holding a plastic implement in her left hand – to wit Exhibit A – commonly known as a vibrator, Your Honour. These women appeared to be in a sexual encounter of sorts. I failed to discern whether they were in a similar state of arousal.'

That didn't happen, of course – not as evidence in the trial at any rate. Maybe it was just as well as it almost certainly would not have lessened the £100 fine and six-month suspended jail sentence handed down to Marion Murphy in relation to brothel-keeping charges at the Kasbah. But the event itself was real. It was a night like many, many nights over ten years and five months when the Kasbah was at its shocking, sizzling and surreal best.

Sitting comfortably in her spacious detached home in a fashionable suburb of Dublin, the trial now a full month behind her, Linda Lavelle looked drained from the whole experience: 'The worst three days of my entire life.' I wondered as I sat there what she thought of me as I made up my mind that she was firmly established in my way of thinking as a friend; someone I'd be happy to do something for just for the sake of it, someone I was quite glad to know and be in the company of, even though I hadn't a dog's idea of what made her tick. She recalled the 'Madhatters' incident with her familiar wicked sense of humour and attention to detail.

'I had one of my Slaves actually put all the metal rings on the ceiling. We had seven of these loopers hitched up to each ring by chains which were connected to their ankles and around their balls, then connected up to the backs of their necks. Imagine if there had been a police raid on one of these nights! I often think about what would have happened then. It would have taken a long time for the police to untie them and take them down to the station. Would they have called in a doctor or a psychologist to help them?'

I was to discover that the night was made even more ghoulishly theatrical by the presence of an eighth client, a British-born businessman living in Ireland for many years now who used the name Marianne, given to him by the girls. He would spend just a few minutes strung from the ceiling before being unchained and allowed to strut around the room proclaiming the size of his organ. 'That was his turn on,' said Linda. 'He needed to hear the girls tell him that he had the biggest cock they'd ever seen. Right enough, he was well hung and he got a buzz out of comparing what he had to the men still hanging out of the ceiling. But he wasn't the biggest the girls had ever seen, not by a long way. It just looked that way because he wasn't such a tall chap.'

The session, prearranged by the men and carried out by the women to the last detail, ends after exactly an hour. One way or another, all the clients attain sexual climax, said Linda. Having done so, their transformation is astonishing, reminding me of the wearily delivered one-liner from Madam Cynthia Payne in the film *Personal Services*: 'A man can't think straight until he's despunked'.

'As soon as they'd come,' Linda told me, 'they'd all get real respectable; go real blushy in the face; want to get out of the room; wouldn't recognise the chap beside them even though they've all been strung out of the fucking ceiling together for the past hour. Then they'd be gone out of the place in two seconds; heads down, back to normality.'

The men at the Kasbah on the night in question, she told me, were students of Frustration. 'It's not quite as extreme as Discipline.'

As she continued talking, it occurred to me for the first time that the thirty-eight-year-old woman sitting on the low sofa opposite me in the front room of her home was at her most relaxed, most affectionate, when talking about these so-called specialist clients. 'They get a turn-on from comparing their cocks with other mens' cocks to see who had the biggest, do you know what I mean? They get a big turn-on from seeing another man being wanked off; to see another man come. On that particular night I sent Mandy in with a vibrator and she was playing with herself on the bed while these loopers were drooling at the mouth watching her, unable to get near their cocks to relieve themselves; they were fucking mad to come! They'd be left like that for an hour. On that particular night Vikki entered the room and simulated sex with Mandy. Then they both got up off the bed and, you know, worked their men, bringing them to the point where they're just about to shoot their load, then they'd back off again. I'd come in from time to time with a cane and let them have it on the arse or the back of the legs and they'd start complaining that one of them didn't get hit as hard as the chap next to him! Frustration is their turn-on. They're not hard Discipline clients at all. They get turned on by tease and frustration – by not having the control to relieve themselves sexually. Would you like some tea or coffee, Dave? Did you have a breakfast yet?'

Not for the first time I asked myself who is this woman before me? Can I believe what she's saying? Why was it that for most of our time together, in her house – on her ground – I felt perfectly at ease, yet when she talked about clients, particularly clients of Discipline and Bondage, I felt utterly confused, both about them and about her. From that early point in March 1993, when the interview stage of research on this book got underway, I started looking for tell-tale signs in Linda Lavelle's psychological make-up that made her say these things and, presumably do these things with men, men she had apparent real feeling for. I didn't realise it at the time, but she was challenging my own preconceived notions about prostitution, about prostitutes: they just had to be fundamentally different from the rest of society, I felt, or they simply would not survive in a world such as theirs. They had to be flawed, emotionally, psychologically or mentally. Either that, or they had fallen into such dire personal straits that they simply had no choice but to sell their bodies to men. Yet here was this woman, this mother and housewife dressed in jeans and a pink *banín* jumper who simply did not fit in with any of these notions.

I thought of those late night calls and the bar-room intelligence depicting her as a hard woman with bags of money. Linda Lavelle is physically very big for a woman, standing at five feet eleven inches and probably weighing about thirteen stone. That presence alone intimidated me at first. It also frightened me in a sexual sense, being one of perhaps many men who are sexually intimidated by big women. But there was nothing hard about Linda that I could detect. Quite the opposite. And if Linda Lavelle is wealthy it is not because she guards her money – she's commonly known as an easy touch for cash among her fellow prostitutes. She is also something of a mother confessor. I was to witness her home being constantly used as a refuge by prostitutes who had found their own domestic or work situations untenable for one reason or another. She is a manager of people rather than a controller of them, an intelligent woman who, I felt, would have made a success out of anything she touched. Right enough, I did find her slightly eccentric and over-the-top – wont to laugh at the oddest of things, particularly the stream of calls coming in on her omnipresent mobile phone through which she directs a nationwide call girl operation in Ireland to this day.

'You want a girl in Galway? Right. Can you wait till Friday, Paddy? You what? Yes, yes, very attractive. Black and young. You what? £150 an hour, Paddy. £100 for half an hour. Is that alright Paddy? Oh, I'm fine. The family's fine, Paddy. Did you sort out the problem with the doctor, Paddy?' She puts her hand over the receiver and giggles as she confides in me. 'Paddy's a nutter. He's got spots on his balls and he wants one of our women to take him to the doctor. It's his fantasy. He's no fucking spots at all, poor man.'

The phone conversation resumes.

'Sure I know it's steep, Paddy. But look at what you're getting. Sure where else would you get a fine looking black girl to ride with lovely breasts for that kind of money. How much have you got, Paddy? [pause] You must be fucking joking me, Paddy! Right. Right, okay. Bye Paddy.' Linda interprets her client for me. 'He's a nice fella. Very highly thought of businessman in the West [of Ireland]. He's been with us for years but he's tight-skinned with money, Dave. He's loaded but he's mean. Yeah, he loves black girls with big boobs. He'll pay once she gets him into the room. He always pays once she gets him into the room.'

Suddenly and without a prompt, Linda corrects herself again. 'Sorry, Dave. You're here for the book and it's getting late again. Who do you think I should start with?'

Chapter Two

'Trust Me . . .'

Linda Lavelle frightened me. I had not yet met her, but intrigue and innuendo followed this woman about the place and for some reason which I couldn't put my finger on, I wished I wasn't in the Clarence Hotel on the Dublin city quaysides waiting on this stranger.

Her name was on the lips of every police officer connected to illicit sex in Dublin right through the 1980s and 1990s. Her name was on the lips of every other prostitute I had interviewed. It was the summer of 1990 and, to both the observers and the practitioners, the world of hired sex in Ireland had become more transparent yet just as steeped in perplexity and taboo as ever.

Thanks to the so-called massage parlours and their extensive carnal menus, the police raids and newspaper exposés, illicit sex had become showbiz in a way which could not have been imagined just a decade earlier when prostitution meant cold dark streets peopled by pitiful women standing in the shadows eyeing the slow moving cars driven by men who were themselves driven by lust, selfishness and emptiness. As a journalist working at the coalface of vice and drugs during that period, I knew that I'd never get the full picture of what was *really* going on behind the headlines and the court cases until I met and gained the confidence of the ubiquitous Ms Lavelle.

Sitting alone in the hotel I recalled the number of times I had received counsel from the police and miscellaneous underworld sources in bar rooms and during night-time telephone calls which went along the lines, 'Do you know the Lavelle one? Linda. Big woman. It's her you should go and see. She's loaded, hard as nails. She's alright, only don't cross her, she could be dangerous, but she'll tell you what's what in the brothel business.'

I had made several phone calls to a place called the Kasbah on Mountjoy Square where everyone knew Ms Lavelle and her ladies operated from. These tentative approaches had taught me at least one lesson that perhaps I should have known already: journalists telephoning massage parlours are by and large wasting their time.

Mullins: I'd like to speak with Linda Lavelle. Is she there?

Kasbah: No, luv. She's not here at the moment. Can I say who's calling?

M: Yeah, Dave Mullins is my name. I'm a reporter and I need to get Linda's side – your side – of the story, of what's going on. Nobody ever writes about it from your side. I'm not trying to do a number on you, I promise.

K: Oh, right luv. And what is it that you think you could do a number on? Would you like to ring back?

M: When?

K: Oh, whenever, luv. Whenever Linda's here, like.

M: And when is that likely to be?

K: Never can tell, luv.

M: Can I look for you? What's your name?

K: Try again later, luv, I've got to be goin. Byeee . . .

One such exasperated call did, however, bear fruit. Halfway through one of many conversations similar to the one above, the voice on the other end changed. This time it was lower in tone. More thoughtful. This time the 'luvs' laced with wariness and misbelief had been replaced by finely measured caution.

Mullins: I'm looking for Linda Lavelle. Hello?

Lavelle: Is that Dave Mullins?

M: Yes

L: This is Linda.

M: Look Linda, I know there are risks in it for you to talk – to trust – someone like me. But I need to talk to you because I'm told you know...

L: Where would you like to meet?

After months of 'Try again later, luv' I had succeeded in setting up the meet. At that moment a feeling of successful journalistic predation forced its way uppermost in my mind and for an instant I forgot that I was still on the phone.

Lavelle: You won't have any photographers with you? Or tape recorders?

Mullins: No, no, no no. Just me. As promised. And it's not an interview and I won't be writing about it in the paper. I just want a meeting. I give you my word.

L: Okay. Right. Say the Clarence Hotel on the quays? What day suits you, Dave?

M: Say Wednesday morning at half-past ten?

L: Okay. You sure you'll be alone?

M: Of course, Linda. I promise you.

L: And you'll write stories the way we see them? That's what you'll do?

M: That's what I would like to do but it's up to you.

L: Right, Dave. I'll see you Wednesday. Bye. Oh, Dave. Are you still there?

M: Yes Linda?

L: Will you make that about twelve o'clock. You know yourself.

A woman such as Linda Lavelle, so connected to and a part of the private lives of so many men, often well-known men, would be invaluable. She was, indeed, a prize journalistic catch. My first thought as I entered the foyer of the Clarence – at that time a middle-of-the-road hotel with regular customers, many from rural Ireland who used it as a stop-off and meeting point from nearby Heuston Station on their journeys to and from Dublin city, was that the character of this old establishment was just right for the type of people I was meeting: transient and inexpensive.

It was just the first of my many prejudices about prostitution, hidden even to myself, to be challenged by the reality.

Linda arrived fifteen minutes late accompanied by a woman I had not heard mention of before whom I will call Pia Masterson. Their entrance into the large bar at the back of the foyer which functioned more as a coffee hall than a pub during daylight hours initially struck me as both arrogant and defiant. Both women were dressed in figure-hugging denims and navy weather-proofed bomber jackets. Both had large black leather handbags anchored to their right shoulders. Somehow I knew that the very tall woman with the shock of natural, free flowing blonde hair and the high, pronounced cheekbones, was the one in charge, was Linda Lavelle. I caught her eye from my seat in the corner and raised a copy of the *Daily Mirror* as if making a bid in an auction room. Neither woman looked at me once as they slowly made their way over to my table.

The talk was of generalities and public attitudes to prostitution. Safe talk with dangerous women, I remembered thinking. References to clients were made in the same vein, except for one hilarious moment when a bespectacled middle-aged man taking tea and biscuits some twenty feet from where we were sitting looked over and spotted Pia and left the premises with such indecent haste that one of his shortbread snaps looked as if it had fallen from the sky onto his chin and shirt collar.

'See that man,' said Pia, the two women enjoying a muffled giggle. 'He's a client of mine and he's just spotted us. He won't be having fucking breakfast in here again!'

On the surface, little or nothing of substance took place: I was given no insight into the world either of these women inhabited that I couldn't have found in a well-written newspaper or magazine feature of the time. Linda Lavelle had come bearing the gifts of potential stories; I had come bearing the promise of discretion and undefined support for the prostitutes. Those were the goods of barter, the vehicles that brought us here. But it was in those other things that happen between people – or sometimes don't happen – beneath the surface and between the words, that left me feeling that the encounter had been a good one. For, there and then, I felt drawn to these two women, particularly to Linda who was already managing to confuse me with her strange facility for caring and mockery at the same time.

I remember driving back to the office and deciding that friendship would be more easily attained with her than trust. I found the notion both dangerous and attractive.

Linda Lavelle only once cryptically referred to the real reason she had taken the risk to meet me. 'There's trouble in the business at the moment, Dave. Do you think you could write a story about a former client who is giving us a lot of trouble? I'll get you all the proof you need. It's a good story for you. Do you think you could expose him?'

Twenty minutes later the two women left by the front door. Things had gone well, I decided. The fact that the meeting took place at all was proof of that. We had made an arrangement to meet again as soon as either of us felt the need to, and the agreement was that no story would be written unless we discussed the matter first. It was Linda's idea that I didn't walk out on to the street with them. She told me later that it was a precaution to prevent me from signalling to a photographer who could have been planted somewhere outside in a parked car. I soon realised that the defiance with which I had earlier accredited them with wasn't that at all. It was fear of a newspaper ambush.

After that point we either met in person or spoke on the phone, at least once a fortnight. Linda regularly called me with background information on vice-related court cases, etc., ending almost every conversation with, 'Jesus, Dave, don't say where you got the information from,' which, after a few months of familiarity, I interpreted as nothing more than a mildly dramatic way of saying cheerio.

I had begun to visit her home – a five-bedroomed detached affair in an exclusive suburb on Dublin's northside. I had suspected that Linda would somehow present a different persona in this place, that she would be in some way distinct from the woman in the hotel once she was within the security of her nest. This was not to be.

I was always invited into the front room, the living room, where Linda would sit on the sofa so as to be able to push the door shut when required with her foot and be close to the phone at the same time. Ellen, her absent-minded maid, served copious amounts tea and cakes brought in from the ranch-style kitchen at the back of the house. Linda confided to me that Ellen wanted to give me a story about the number of abortions she had had but was too shy. 'Would you run a story like that? She [Ellen] thinks she might be pregnant again. She's not sure but she thinks one of her neighbours from the southern end of the country is the father. The poor oul creature can't manage. I have her here out of charity. She's not fit to be a maid, she's no fucking good at it but she thinks she's the bee's knees! Would you be interested in things like that, Dave?'

Once distracted from interviews, Linda would talk about the people in this, her other life: about her long-time companion, Liam (not his real name); her sons aged nineteen and twenty-one and her daughters, aged sixteen and six. It was a

small talk that I found disturbing only because it was so familiar, so normal: the sort of talk you'd hear in any home in
Ireland which housed a near-grown-up family. The state of her
home was also familiar. I had expected brash attempts at
ostentation and perhaps vague signs of vulgarity, of her
wealth – deep pink carpet piles and satin curtains from ceiling
to floor, that sort of thing. It was nothing like that, just a
plain and lived-in home. The front room where I conducted
the interviews owed more to function than aestheticism: there
was a twenty-three-inch television in a corner with the
inevitable video recorder underneath it. Large photographic
portraits of her four children hung on the wall housing the
chimney. Hers are strong children, healthy and handsome.
Underneath the pictures, the fireplace had become a still-life
thanks to a coal-effect gas fire. A black leather suite of furniture that had seen better days dominated the room. A wooden
coffee table with a mosaic inlay in the centre of the floor
always prompted Linda's warning, 'Be careful of the leg, Dave,
the leg on that should have been fixed years ago.'

Only two fixtures were out of the ordinary. One was the
large red curtain draping the back wall of the room. I was certain, although I don't know why, that there were no doors or
windows in the wall and its presence seemed appropriately
odd. The other fixture was the large oak bar in the corner of
the square room which resided at a tilt as though one of the
castors was missing and which always reminded me of an old
wooden ship that had run aground. This now unused booze
depot would, I guessed, have owed more to its existence to
Liam than to Linda.

'I come back from work in Cork and the place is like a pig
sty. I'll tell you, Dave, they'd all be in the poorhouse it if wasn't
for me. Liam won't lift a finger to tidy the place. Never has, the
fucker. At least the two lads have never been in any trouble at
school or anywhere else. Thank God for that.'

At another, later time, Linda spoke about her eldest son

being turfed out of school for wearing the wrong shoes too often. She said she has bought him special shoes 'fashion shoes', she described them, £120 per pair and three pairs in the past twelve months. 'Wait until you get them [my children] to their ages,' she told me. 'They'll really cause you hassle and heartache then.'

In this context she told the story of her nineteen-year-old son who once asked whether he and a pal could have a couple of cans of beer that were stocked in the house during Christmas as they wanted to stay in and watch a couple of videos. 'I only allowed them both one can of beer each,' she said. 'I mean, what's a parent supposed to do? Are we to say "no" and have them drinking cider in the fields just because they want to taste booze? They'd do it one way or the other whether you let them or not so I thought it was better that he had a drink in the house where nothing too bad could go wrong. Boy, was I wrong about that. I went to bed early and much later I heard John [not his real name] slip on the stairs. I shouted down "What's wrong?" and he said "Nothing, Mam, you stay where you are." When he said that I knew there was something wrong and I came downstairs. Well, Dave, I've never . . . my fella was drunk but he wasn't too bad but the other fella was sprawled all over the back garden getting as sick as a pregnant pig. It's just as well that an ambulance was called because he had to get his stomach pumped out in hospital and I heard later he could have killed himself if he hadn't vomited.

'The two little bastards had drank a couple of bottles of brandy I'd got in for the Christmas. In one hour they'd got through the fucking lot and after it was all over my lad even had the neck to suggest that I'd let him drink it! I was left without a drop of brandy in the house all over the Christmas and John was blaming me for letting him drink it! At least the other fellow, when he got out of hospital, had the good manners and rearing to come around to my house and apologise.'

*

Once during research interviews at Linda's home which were always carried out before lunchtime when her children would be in school, she invited me to a Discipline session involving a client who would pay £1,000 each to five prostitutes to be whipped in a specially kitted out sex dungeon in one of her several privately owned buildings. She believed that if I could covertly witness the event I would get a better feel for the writing of the book. 'He'll be tied to a pole with black paint all over his balls and penis,' she said, 'I'll be the one doing the whipping.'

After picking up on my apprehension at such an invitation, Linda assured me, 'you've nothing to be frightened of, Dave. Even if he spots you he won't go near you. He'll do as I tell him when he's in role. He'll fucking well bark and eat his own shite if I tell him to.'

Naturally, I refused her invitation. In an effort to hide my inability to accept and embarrassment at being asked along, I half jokingly enquired whether she would ensure that the paint was non-toxic and quite matter-of-factly she replied that she would raid her younger daughter's art box in the bedroom for the paint while Ellen kept the child downstairs, and put it back the following morning before she could notice it was gone.

Breakfast time at Linda's house, I resolved from an early point in my visits, was an event I was not meant to ever fully understand.

From time to time Linda would remind me of why she had agreed to meet me in the first place, although she never put it that bluntly. 'When are you going to expose Little John? Remember I told you about Little John. Youse did a story on him already. Do you want to meet him? I'll get him to talk to you. He's a bit of a nutter but he'll talk if you want him to.'

My journalistic colleague Eddie Rowley had already interviewed 'Little John' Keegan – about how he spent all of his Post Office redundancy money on a prostitute who blew him out when the money was all gone – and other newspapers in the city subsequently ran with a similar story, although Keegan was not identified in the newspapers until later. I told Linda I needed a new angle on the story; I needed to name Little John and I didn't think it was legally safe to do so at the time.

It was then that she revealed that Keegan had gone to the police with his story of the prostitutes at the Kasbah by way of an official complaint. She desperately wanted him stopped in his tracks and asked me straightforwardly whether I could help. 'This is going to end up in court, Dave. That fucker Keegan is going to put us all out of business. The police are already beginning to ask questions. They are taking his complaints very seriously. Oh, Jesus, he's going to put us all in jail.'

As we sat drinking coffee in the Clarence Hotel and in her almost stately home during those mornings in the late summer of 1991, one full year after we had first met, an unmarked police van containing several officers and video recording equipment was already in place on the opposite side of the road to 60B Mountjoy Square West – the Kasbah – and around the corner outside a similar basement premises at 24 Belvedere Place.

As the weeks passed leading up to Christmas there was much more alcohol and urgency about the hotel coffee mornings. Linda brought other women with her besides Pia Masterson. For the first time in my company, the teas, coffees and biscuits were being replaced by large brandies, Scotches and vodkas. More cigarettes were smoked. The agenda was no longer Little John Keegan but Marion Murphy: the woman in whose name the Kasbah was leased. She had guessed rightly that she was about to be charged with managing and keeping a brothel at both the Kasbah and Belvedere Place – Laura's Studio – and word had it that she was going to plead not guilty to all counts. Mandy Jameson, Charlene Robertson, Georgina O'Kane, Vikki O'Toole (not real names) and other prostitutes seemed ambivalent about Marion Murphy's decision to contest the charges. These were frightened women. They figured Marion was right in moral terms but no one knew better than they that right decisions and wrong decisions didn't look after the bills and their game, above all games, was about making good money and steering clear of the law often at great cost to themselves.

I was given a new role by the women as something of an unofficial legal adviser. Yet I saw little point in imparting any expertise I might have had because I could see that Linda and some of the other prostitutes I had met at the Kasbah wanted to see the legal processes through, no matter what I or anyone else had to say. Marion Murphy herself figured that a guilty plea leading to automatic conviction, while not ruinous, would leave her vulnerable to subsequent litigation which could land her in jail. (She already had a vice record – a conviction for prostitution back in 1977 which required an overnight stay in Mountjoy jail, an institution not a stone's throw away from the Kasbah.)

But there were other factors steeling the resolve of the more resilient prostitutes of the Kasbah which went way beyond the dynamics of the upcoming trial and the concern it was causing to a handful of prostitutes privy to all the details: it was Linda Lavelle's belief, for example, that someone in the vice business would sooner or later have to take a stand against the police. Brothels fronting as massage parlours had been the subject of fairly intensive police scrutiny since the early 1980s when thirty-eight sex-rub joints were known to be operating in the city of Dublin. And, even though the cops themselves had little stomach for annoying prostitutes and their clients, they had no option but to do so when formal complaints were made against the premises, usually by disgruntled neighbours. Once in court, the girls would invariably plead guilty to brothel-keeping in the usually sound knowledge that such a course of action would earn them a relatively small fine and the dreaded evidence from clients would not be required by the State to prove its case.

In one sense it was the best of both worlds: the police would have their conviction; the complaining neighbour would have his sense of indignation vindicated; and the Madams, while closed down by the raid, usually set up shop in a different location soon after conviction, their reputation for confidentiality affirmed in the eyes of their grateful clients. The whole business was, of course, inherently unfair and it was this ideological injustice which vexed Linda Lavelle and other 'management' prostitutes so much. 'Why the fuck should we take all the stick? Why should we be the ones fined, jailed, and identified all the time? What about the clients? These powerful bastards who are never charged or identified?'

Of course she was right. Nowhere is grim patriarchy more evident in Ireland than in the area of paid sex, and by sticking to her pleas of not guilty despite informal advice to the contrary from some well-meaning members of the police force and from a section of prostitutes around the city who were understandably more interested in maintaining their own salvation, Marion Murphy was lighting a powder keg under that very same deep-rooted patriarchal condition: for the first time in the modern history of the State, the prospect of clients to a bordello being identified in a public arena was a very real one.

The first public whiff of scandal surrounding the Kasbah surfaced in the national press in late August 1991 when it was leaked that an eminent Irish political figure had been caught on a police surveillance video entering and leaving a bordello in Dublin city along with a Gaelic Athletic Association (GAA) (Ireland's largest native sporting institution) man, a publican, and other well-known men. As it turned out, the politician in question declined police invitations to make a statement about his movements, so to speak, offering only the legally required minimum name-rank-and-serial-number drill. There was never any possibility, therefore, of him appearing in open court to give evidence against Marion Murphy, a scenario some newspapers mistakenly salivated over for weeks. (For the record, the politician has been a client of the Kasbah for the past ten years. He continues to take 'Discipline classes' from Linda and the girls to this very day. The Monday after the Circuit Criminal Court found Marion Murphy guilty, he telephoned Linda offering sympathy, encouragement and support, and seeking an appointment for sex.)

The clients who elected at that time to give full statements of their experiences at either the Kasbah or Laura's Studio did so in the belief that, while they might later be called to give evidence, they would in all probability not be named or identified. Not to give statements, the police told them at the time, could result in detectives calling at their home in the course of their investigations.

All but two of the men were married.

It was only by dint of good fortune and an agreement between Judge Buchanan and counsel for both Defence and State, which was not binding on journalists, that the thirteen witnesses, some of them important figures in Irish life including the man referred to in the newspapers at the time as 'the leading GAA man', remained only as Witness A, B, C, and so forth, during the trial and in media reports.

The excitement for me was very real, being as I was the only journalist to know exactly what was going on and to have in my possession the names and addresses of the clients concerned. I knew, also, that the depositions they had signed in the lower courts admitting to sexual services in the Kasbah and presumably made in a desperate attempt to shield their secret lives from their families, bore little resemblance to what the prostitutes serving them claimed they were seeking, and getting, from the women of the bordello. But the big, and still unbroken, story was, of course, the publication of the identity of the politician who frequented the Kasbah. I had known for some time previous to the courtroom drama who the individual was. The question whether to name the clients who signed the depositions, and the politician the whole political and journalistic community in Dublin was talking about at the time, was constantly raised at newsroom meetings in the *Sunday World* where I worked and, presumably, within the editorial confines of other newspaper offices in the city and across the water in Britain.

The ethical question of naming the politician threw up the old arguments of the public's right to know as opposed to the personal privacy of the individual – even if that individual was and is a public figure. I don't know where to draw that fine line, and I get more confused when I hear the issue being debated publicly and read the guidelines set down to help journalists make such decisions. The principle that the private affairs of a public figure should become public knowledge at the point where the police take a part in the proceedings is, for instance, often used as a bench mark for journalistic interference. Personally, I would prefer to remain confused than to hand across such power to the police or anyone else for that matter. As it was, I felt that naming the politician who frequented the massage parlour in this case was gratuitously nasty and I let myself be guided by this instinct.

But the solution wasn't that simple. By knowing the politician's identity and deciding not to reveal it, the newspaper I worked for was running the risk of being 'scooped' by the competition. Already, the Irish editions of some of the British tabloids had gone further than other newspapers by revealing the politician's precise office: it was a clear signal to their rivals that the gloves were off and names could imminently find their way into print.

As it happened, the politician's identity remained, if not unknown, then at least spared from becoming part of the public domain. I had two reactions to that event. Firstly, I had the feeling that the right thing had been done, or, at least, that the wrong thing hadn't been done and that this man and his family had been spared the public ignominy of his being seen, on the one hand, as a respected public figure with authority and leadership and at the same time as a client of prostitutes operating a bordello catering to the most extreme demands of sexual desire.

But there was also the feeling of being cheated. I had spent an enormous amount of time and effort getting to the point where I could safely (from a legal point of view) publicly expose this individual and now, with the end of my investigative race clearly in sight, I wasn't getting the pay-off, *my* pay-off. I have spent nearly fifteen years of my life pursuing the type of stories where the public's right to know is blindingly obvious but which, primarily for legal reasons, never see the light of day. To have a major story shelved on any grounds, including those of principle, is not uncommon, just extremely difficult because it goes against the training.

Then there was Linda Lavelle, her words still echoing inside me. 'Why the fuck should we take all the stick? Why should we be the ones fined, jailed, and identified all the time? What about the clients? These powerful bastards who are never charged or identified?' By not identifying the politician and the other clients in this book I have, to some degree, parted from Linda Lavelle's original motivation for the project. I don't have answers to her questions. And I don't have a solution to this dilemma, just the strongly held belief that this is a story of Irish women and men that should be told and that their story is far more important than the identity of their clients.

The three days of Marion Murphy's trial caused considerable public confusion and irritation – if not anger. As a journalist covering the case for the *Sunday World*, many people asked me how such an event could take up the time and resources of the Irish police force – the Garda Síochána – when the country remained in the throes of a serious crime wave, particularly in the areas of family violence, armed crime and drug abuse. The belief that the population would have been better served with every available police officer committed to these tasks rather than rounding up a thirty-eight-year-old mother of four who ran a grotty little sex den for perverts was, and still, is widespread.

There was also disquiet with more psychological undertones, particularly among men and voiced only in safe moments: that clandestine sex was under threat as never before in Ireland. Bishop Eamonn Casey hadn't escaped his particular weaknesses and now these clients to the massage parlours had come to the precipice of public humiliation and personal ruin. Safe sex, in the widest sense of the term, had suddenly become an extremely rare commodity.

In truth, the police had little choice but to deliver Marion Murphy and her vice operations to the scrutiny of the judicial system, thanks to a man who remained faceless throughout her trial and whose very existence was only briefly referred to in the final hour of the three-day hearing. John Keegan, a deluded but highly intelligent former Post Office worker, had conducted a wantonly vengeful campaign against the prostitutes of Mountjoy Square and Belvedere Place and in so doing, had unwittingly changed the shape of prostitution in Ireland – much for the worse as far as the women who inhabit that world are concerned.

From the first time we spoke about the matter, Marion Murphy was determined to enter not guilty pleas to the upcoming charges of keeping and managing brothels at both premises. She would do so on the mistaken assumption that there was insufficient evidence to link her directly with the knowledge that both businesses were being run as anything other than bona fide massage parlours where paid-for sexual services, to use her own words to the police at the time, were 'definitely not' on offer.

Keegan, who basked in the self-bestowed title of The Inch-high Private Eye, formally complained to the police and, by extension, to the Garda Commissioner; he even went so far as to report what he guessed were Marion Murphy's earnings to the Revenue Commissioners. A senior police figure told me during the trial, 'It's not that hard to understand why all this is happening. The type of complaints and detailed information we got from Keegan meant we had to act: not to do so would have left us open to accusations of corruption and complicity from every conceivable quarter.'

Back in the living room of Linda Lavelle's home two months after the trial nothing much had changed for her in a material sense. She was still 'looking after' men; she is as busy as ever, but still found all the time I needed from her to help me with the book, although no longer motivated on a personal level. 'Lesson One,' she says, 'once a pervert, always a pervert and Kasbah or no Kasbah they'll never go away. And neither will I. I'm in this business for life because I choose to be. I wouldn't work at anything else.'

Over the following months Linda Lavelle, ably assisted by the women who still worked for and with her, took me on a journey through the lives of her women and their men clients. 'We'll talk about the Slaves first,' she says, 'because they're very interesting nutters altogether!' She explained that the term 'Slave' is applied by the prostitutes to men from all walks of life who live out their fantasies of often absurd and infantile subservience to their chosen 'Mistresses' – the name usually applied to the women who worked at the Kasbah and who were only too willing to metamorphose into whatever persona or role was required of them by these strange, yet outwardly normal, men.

Theirs is a story which includes the kinky sexual adventures of three errant and powerful Roman Catholic churchmen, two of whom were regular Kasbah clients and are still using former Kasbah girls to this day. Many TDs (members of the Irish Parliament), including the notorious politician dubbed by the girls as The Fat-Assed Slave were, and still are, clients to the women of the Kasbah. Scores of priests have visited what many would regard as this most sinful of places over the years, their confessions now told by their women servers. Senior and rank-and-file members of the police force were among the Kasbah's most enduring clients, including the highly thought of officer who drove naked through Dublin's city centre for all-night sex in the infamous Hellfire Club, situated high in the surrounding Dublin Mountains where, lore has it, the Devil appeared in cloven feet during a card game. There is Smelly Bottoms, the well-known actor who delights in the atrocities of scatology – sexual excitement through the use of human excrement.

And there is, of course, the strange story of Little John Keegan, the 'dotty little brothel creeper who fucked up everything for us' and his obsession with Margaret 'Poppy' Healy, the prostitute who, as a barmaid in a County Cork hotel, befriended Bishop Eamonn Casey before she turned to a life of vice, and who had an affair with Keegan for as long as his £12,000 nest egg held out.

Above all, there is the Kasbah and Linda Lavelle and the incredible world she and her girls kneaded out of the minds and bodies of men in the heart of a nation's capital city.

It is a world that almost survived. The Kasbah is no more, and this time it is not likely to undergo one of its occasional rebirths. But the events that went on there are now chronicled for the first time, for all time.

Chapter Three

The Life And Death Of John Bones

It was probably the biggest day of John Bones's life. He had prepared himself well: a double course of Vivioptal vitamins and iron washed down with three glasses of sherry every night for a month; a diet of rare liver and fresh vegetables; bed by 7pm. He had shed a few pounds, although still a respectable sixteen and a half stones held together by a wiry but ample six foot frame. An unaccustomed four weeks of self-enforced celibacy ensured that he was in peak condition.

That morning he shaved, donned his best pinstripe suit, complete with red rose in his left lapel, before making his way slowly to Dublin in his battered green vintage Morris Minor. The farm would have to survive without him for one day at least. After all, wasn't he attending the serious business of ensuring an heir to the holding? By 11am, he had made his way off the motorway, through the south city suburb of Harold's Cross before chugging into the city centre, a pair of bell-bottom jeans wrapped neatly into a paper parcel on the passenger seat beside him – his gift to a woman he knew only as Jan. Bones would never park his car closer than 500 yards from his destination, the basement of 60B Mountjoy Square West. He was, by all accounts, a cautious man by birth and by nature, and a figure held in some authority and respect in the tightly knit rural community where he had lived all his life.

He had known Jan and Linda for over a decade, being a regular client to the house in Harold's Cross Road which both women had used as a brothel in the late 1970s and early 1980s. He was one of a legion of men who had continued their patronage when the two women set up massage parlours in Mountjoy Square in the early 1980s. And like so many of them, he had developed a one-sided infatuation for the women. In the case of John Bones (Bones was a nickname given him by Linda), he had fallen for both women and was quite convinced that they felt the same way about him. Bones's feelings were affirmed when Jan agreed to have his child. He never twigged that he was just one of many clients who became the butt of malevolent wind-ups in a profession where the line between being paid for abetting fantasy and engaging in the cruellest of ridicule is often blurred.

A month earlier, sad John Bones had asked Linda whether she would be interested in having his baby. 'We were just talking away after a session,' she recalled. 'He paid me the money and I asked him casually whether he had any children. The lying bastard said "no" although I now know he was a grandfather. I knew from experience what was coming next. He just stared at me and said quietly, "Would you like to have a child by me, Linda?" I said I couldn't possibly do that because of a relationship I was in but I knew that Jan was anxious to have a child and John Bones said, "I'd be very glad to oblige. I just want to be a father, Linda."

'Can you just fucking well imagine that!'

Linda continued, 'I told Jan what was going on and she was game. The next week she sized Bones up when he came in for his usual grope and a ride. "You're perfect for me," she said. "You've got blue eyes and you're tall like me. I'd love to have your baby, John."'

If Farmer John was delighted he didn't show it. Perhaps deals are deals and a man of the earth rarely shows his inner responses. 'Right,' he told Jan Tyler (not her real name) with post-coital ease, 'I'll be back in a month and we'll have a go at it then.' He made an appointment for a Friday morning four weeks hence and walked off to his trusty Morris parked somewhere in the rush-hour of the urban ant colony. 'He was wearing the same farm-work clothes he always wore when he visited massage parlours,' recalled Jan. 'John visited a lot of parlours and it was always the same story – he was dressed just like he came in out of the fields after a day's work pulling spuds.'

Neither Linda nor Jan knew quite how their gentle giant had received their farcical invitation. They didn't much care, either: in the world of prostitution, I discovered, survival depends on the ability to expect and cope with the unexpected. But even this pair of street-wise ladies could not have foreseen that, later rather than sooner, something uniquely and dreadfully special would happen in the case of John Bones.

By the summer of 1988, the 'rival' massage parlours of the two former one-room hookers from Harold's Cross, both situated on Mountjoy Square, couldn't keep up with demand. Two years earlier Linda even opened a second premises in nearby 24 Belvedere Place (her tenancy of number 44 on the same street was short-lived after the landlord there learnt what was going on and promptly advised her of her limited options for staying clear of the processes of law) and was fast becoming well off.

Linda's Kasbah was by this stage the best-known whorehouse in the country and the then thirty-six-year-old Ms Lavelle had already established herself as the uncrowned queen of vice in Ireland. She had come a long way from jointly running a seedy little south city knocking shop on Harold's Cross Road – putting up with complaints from neighbours about the queues of men on the footpath outside at all hours of the day and night waiting anxiously to sample the delights of both herself and Jan. In the 1970s she had lived with her companion Liam (and for a short while their new baby son) high in the Dublin Mountains in a Fiat 124 S rust bucket that provided them with both transport and shelter during their initial days in the city in search of work and money and the fulfilment of undefined dreams.

It was the ability to extract advantage from adversity that gave Linda Lavelle the idea of setting up a purpose-built brothel: no complaints from neighbours, no queues, and money for the asking. Well, almost for the asking. What she had also begun, perhaps unknown to herself at the time, was a revolution in the paid sex business in Ireland. 'The 1970s thing was all street stuff and it was dangerous,' she often told me. 'The massage parlours brought in a new era, with better conditions, better money and a safer way of making it.'

When, on 20 May 1981, the Kasbah opened its doors for the first time, it wasn't the first sex-rub joint fronting as a massage parlour in town to do so, but it was certainly a far cry from the myriad grotty little city-centre dens run by one or two over-aged and often drink-troubled women, controlled by pimps and offering little more than straight sex and masturbation. From day one, the Kasbah was different. In the words of Vikki, one of its most endearing and fractious women, it was 'a place of total whores' where anything and everything was on the menu. And, perhaps most importantly for the girls who worked there, it was controlled by women, prostitute women at that.

John Bones arrived at the pre-arranged time on the Friday morning after his four-weeks' training for the first step in his revisitation of fatherhood. He was met by Linda who was taken aback by his lean and polished countenance; the suit, the red rose in the lapel and the mysterious brown paper parcel under his oxter. Her mind was racing. What the fuck was she going tell him? 'Girls don't do it without condoms unless they're planning a child and sure as fuck Jan ain't planning no child by you, John Bones, no matter how fucking dickied up and washed you are.' For the first time in her years of serving him, she became aware of Bones's physical bulk. He wouldn't be the first client she'd come to blows with but, she thought as she looked up into his eyes, he might be her last.

'I'm very sorry, John,' she started off. 'Jan isn't well at the moment. You'll have to come back another day.'

Her lies didn't impress. Bones blew up. 'I have spent a fortune getting myself prepared for this day. It is the biggest day of my life. It has to be done today.'

Anxiety crept into his voice and Linda felt marginally less threatened. 'I'll never be in this condition again, don't you see? I'll never be able to give her the baby she wants from me. It's got to be today.' Linda recalled her thoughts at that moment: 'Is this man totally off his rocker?' She continued her lies. 'She's in hospital, John. She has one of those women's complaints. Boils on her . . . she's going to have a hysterectomy. Try and understand.'

John Bones didn't have time to absorb any of it. His wrinkled but handsome face had turned from bemusement to disbelief as, over Linda's shoulder, he caught sight of Jan Tyler walking towards them in apparent rude health, tears of laughter streaming down her face after witnessing Linda desperately trying to crawl out of the hole she had dug for herself. Bones became angrier than before and boomed at Linda, 'Now you have Jan crying. Are you happy now, you selfish pig.' He was spitting out the words nose-to-nose, eyeball-to-eyeball at Linda who decided at that point that reasoned deceit no longer offered adequate protection. She turned her back and legged it down the street, leaving Bones to comfort one quite hysterically amused hooker.

John Bones eventually got the message that it had all been some sort of cruel joke with him as the victim. He refused to talk to Linda for months, choosing correctly but for all the wrong reasons, to blame her for everything. It didn't stop him from his weekly visits to the Kasbah. In fact, he ended his days there, pathetically falling in love again, this time with Margaret 'Poppy' Healy. It was while he was smack bang wallop in the middle of riding Poppy that he suffered a massive and fatal heart attack. The newspapers of the day carried a two-paragraph 'filler' recording that a man, whom they did not identify, had died in 'one of the city's better known massage parlour sex dens.'

The death of John Bones had, in fact, developed into a full-blown crisis at the Kasbah for Linda and the other women who were on duty that day. She recalled, 'Old Bones was going hell-for-leather on top of Poppy on the bed when suddenly she screamed out for me. I ran in and she had just managed to get out from underneath him. She was crying on about hearing him make some sort of croaking sound. I said to her not to be stupid; he's always playing games. She told me she had seen the look of death in his eye just before he collapsed and she just managed to get out from underneath him in time. It would have been tough fucking luck for her if she hadn't. Imagine having sixteen stone of dead man on top of you and inside you at the same time!'

It was the first time anyone had died in the Kasbah and the first time a young prostitute called Helen (not her real name) had to take a condom and two erection rings (elasticated bands of rubber tied at the base of the penis and around the scrotum, applied for the purpose of enhancing and prolonging an erection) off a dead man. Linda headed down to nearby Fitzgibbon Street police station to inform them of an emergency as the phone in the Kasbah was prudently rigged for incoming calls only. Bones's death in October 1989 would mark the first of many visits she would make to police stations over the coming two years. She informed the young female officer behind the perspex screen that a man was after dying in 60B Mountjoy Square – 'the Kasbah, dear' – and could the police organise an ambulance? When she got back she found Poppy still in the room, sitting in a corner stark naked and bawling her eyes out. The ambulance men were preparing two plastic bags: one for the still-naked corpse of John Bones and the other for his belongings, which included trousers, socks, shirt, and shoes stacked neatly on a table beside the bed, crowned with two sets of false teeth, one still glistening in its wetness. The medics had earlier tried in vain to resuscitate Bones and created a great deal of noise in the process. Helen remembered, 'The noise [sic] blew the light bulbs and the whole place was in pitch dark. It was really scary and I can remember hearing Linda shouting as the ambulance men called for light, "Fuck it, that's all we need, the Devil's in here now. Poppy! Poppy! Can you hear me Poppy? – Shut the fuck up crying and get dressed will you."'

Bones was taken away and given a decent burial by his family. The whole affair stayed 'decent' thanks to a number of policemen who managed through skilful and sensitive paperwork to conceal the exact location of his expiry from this world. To this day the ones who loved and lived with John Bones had no idea what his weekly trips to Dublin were all about. His nephews and nieces spent two days walking the streets of Dublin before they recovered his car.

A police contact later told me that, back at the farm some weeks later, one of John Bones's nephews gave the old motor a long-overdue clean-out and came across a neat brown paper parcel in the boot containing a pair of woman's bell-bottom trousers. It didn't go any further in solving the mystery.

Part at least of the money Bones had given to Poppy Healy that day for his last and apparently thundering ride on this planet found its way into the palm of a young priest in nearby Gardiner Street church. Poppy had made one of her regular excursions into the House of God, this time to have a Mass said 'for a dear departed friend'. There was no irreverence in her choice of words: Poppy frequently spoke in such strange and inappropriate terms of endearment. That night as she sat in the Old Triangle public house with Linda and Vikki and Helen and some of the other girls, surveying the wreckage of a very strange day, Poppy Healy consoled herself that at least Bones had died a happy man, God rest him.

Chapter Four

Oh, Happy Days!

Even Linda Lavelle, with all her entrepreneurial insight into sex
and money, could not have envisaged that some of the cream of
Irish life would one day soon visit this place as she precariously
surveyed the filth and shambles from the top of a makeshift
wooden ladder. From a hole in the ground-level floor above,
through which the ladder descended, her good friend and long-
time client, Tim Rogers (not his real name), was nattering on
about the 'great potential' of the place as the twin vile odours of
vomit and human excrement from the two large rooms below
filled Linda's nostrils. Tim dabbled in the property business
from time to time and had happened upon this premises
through a friend in the trade. 'He was barely able to contain
his excitement,' said Linda. She was barely able to contain the
contents of her stomach.

Empty bottles of cheap Valpariso cooking sherry were
exposed by a single shaft of light entering from a huge hole
constructed out of desperation in the back wall leading out
into the tiny courtyard. And there was sound coming from
this cess pit below. Linda and Tim's presence had prematurely
nudged a few winos from their usual comatose state to the
living hell of dehydrated semiconsciousness. Two of the down-
and-outs decided to share the experience with the blurred

figure of Linda atop the ladder, telling her to get the fuck away if she knew what was good for her.

Linda remembers thinking to herself at the time, 'There must be something wrong with your head if you want to manage this fucking place.'

But she was impressed by the talk from the affable scholar. 'Tim was the type of man who did not hide the fact that he had been in loads of brothels,' said Linda. 'He talked about converting the place into one big room and loads of little rooms with a few nice young birds in little mini skirts beside a roaring log fire waiting to bring their clients into the little rooms.' She adopted his plans and would later tone down the lighting at his suggestion.

A very short time later Marion Murphy took tenancy of the basement of 60B Mountjoy Square West when she signed a lease agreement with a man called Noel O'Gara who subsequently came to some public prominence when he wrote a book about his former buddy, Billy Treacy, accusing him of being the real Yorkshire Ripper. A copy of a lease agreement countersigned by O'Gara on 20 November 1982, and relating to the basement at 60B Mountjoy Square West, and also signed by Vicki Collins (Marion Murphy) and another called Janet Mullins, names O'Gara – an accountant born in Athlone, County Westmeath – as the lessor, although there is nothing to suggest that he had any interest in, or knowledge of, what went on in the Kasbah.

The Kasbah Health and Fitness Studio opened its doors for business for the first time on 20 May 1981. Thanks to Tim Rogers's advice and Linda Lavelle's natural insight into the extremes of male sexuality, it was instantly acknowledged as 'alternative' in nature – both by clients and by the girls who worked there. And it made waves from the very first day, when a leading diplomat got out of his bullet-proof limousine and started taking pictures of his very good friend, Linda, on the footpath outside the new 'Health Studio' she managed and had partly financed: all this much to the confusion of an elderly traffic warden who received a crash-course on diplomatic immunity, its effects on international trade and the man in the street by an equally diplomatic but firm-handed chauffeur.

The name 'Kasbah' only appeared on judicial and police reports and in magazine advertisements. Just three characters affixed to the wall behind the railings – a brass '6' a '0', and a letter 'B' hanging at an angle from its lower mounting, identified 60B Mountjoy Square West from among the grey rows of mostly run-down Georgian buildings, once citadels of the class-conscious professional elite in an age long since gone.

Once inside, however, the Kasbah was quite exquisitely and uniquely decadent. 'Exactly want a man wants' in the words of its celebrated Madam, Linda Lavelle.

A large dimly lit room opens up through the steel-reinforced black door at the bottom of the iron steps. Yellow, red and dark pink bulbs glow around the place like large, irradiated mushrooms mixing with the slow music to create a kind of moody soporific cocktail. An expensive bottle-green velvet curtain hangs from the ceiling dividing the room in half and stops an inch shy of the hotel-standard carpet of red, black and grey stripes. From behind the curtain come the muffled sounds of women talking, laughing, whispering. Three of them are sitting on a sofa made up of the same colours as the carpet. Two are smoking cigarettes and wearing see-through blouses. The amber flames from the coal fire ricochet off the high-gloss finish of the red skirting boards. One of the women looks young, perhaps in her late teens, although it is hard to tell in the light. The other two are older. All three of them have discarded their shoes. They curl up their toes and giggle at the punch-line to a joke with the naïve intimacy of schoolgirls discussing the shortcomings of a shared boyfriend. The younger woman's black leather mini-skirt rides an inch up her thigh as she laughs.

She spots you and it is her call.

She nods silently to the others and walks over to where you're standing. 'Hi,' she says. 'My name is Pam [not her real name]. Can I do anything for you?' If it's your first time she'll know that instinctively. ('It's one of the first things you learn in this game – the new ones. Nervous men can be right fucking trouble,' Vikki O'Toole had once told me.) Pam leads you behind the bottle-green curtain and down a narrow hallway off the big room where she had been sitting, three brown doors with red trimmings on the left, two on the right. At the bottom of the hall hangs a solitary picture depicting a white swan, its outspanned wing protecting a male nude with its long neck and beak curling around to the genitals.

The carpets are the same, so are the shocking red skirting boards, but it seems even more dimly lit than before. She brings you to a room not much bigger than an economy class cabin on a passenger ferry. There are mirrors on the walls and on the artificially low ceiling. A sort of modern-art picture of erotica sits above the freshly dressed single bed. The mood music is still playing and there's a locker beside the bed containing body lotion, talcum powder, baby oil, a white full-length towel. A lamp gives off just a glow of light, a red glow, of course. A twelve-inch television is mounted in the angle at the ceiling. On the floor directly underneath it is a video recorder; on top of it is a black plastic cassette box bearing the words *Huge Bras Number 4* scrawled in biro. The girl calling herself Pam invites you to get undressed and asks for the £15 'book money' – the minimum admission charge and the method by which the Madam makes her living. You're left alone for about ten minutes to prepare yourself.

The girl comes back and asks whether you want any 'extras' – a euphemism for sexual services. Money is always paid up front, unless payment itself constitutes part of the fantasy. The money for the extras goes straight to the prostitute and varies depending on what is being offered and how much money she thinks she can wheedle out of you. While Pam is outside waiting she'll check whether there are any clients using the sauna. If so, she'll put on a spectacular performance for her own client, knowing that she's being observed by at least one other man. For the sauna in the Kasbah was rarely used for the purpose for which it was designed. Rather, it was known by several voyeuristic clients as 'The Peephole'. A recurring band of men would regularly pay £100 a time to see live sex through a knot-hole in the wood, ingeniously engineered by Linda. 'The girl always knew when she was being watched,' she said. 'And the client never, never knew.' The girls did not receive extra payments for these audience friendly performances. One can only surmise that a combination of sexual ego and professional pride was motivation enough for their calorie-burning specials on such occasions.

These were the very best of times for Linda Lavelle, financially at least. She had come a long way from slumming it with her long-time partner Liam in the foothills of the Dublin Mountains living in a banged-out Fiat 124 Sports, broke with little else but their dreams, making meals on a camping gas placed in the rear of the car and using water from a nearby public hand pump. By then their seven-month-old baby son was in the care of Linda's mother far away in a Border county farm. That was in the spring of 1973.

Linda and Liam had met a few years earlier in Wexford where she worked waitressing in a hotel and where he was foreman on a building site. Marriage was always out, Liam was already hitched but that fire didn't last. From the moment they met, however, they were a team. They are still a team today even if it is sometimes impossible, for me at least, to imagine how such a relationship could work.

With an idealism belonging mostly to the young, they had decided at an early point to leave the limiting confines of their rural base and head for the Big Smoke of Dublin to make their mark. Liam had ideas of setting up his own construction business and, with a woman as strong as Linda behind him, he knew that anything was possible. They spent their first six weeks high in the mountains over looking this city of promise. They were often cold, often hungry. I suspect that her view of things was always more realistic than his sense of optimism and it wasn't long before the young Ms Lavelle started coming down from the mountains two or three nights every week . . .

At first Liam didn't know what to make of his woman's nocturnal outings. Linda would always get a taxi back to within fifty yards of their 'mobile home' and walk the rest of the way, but it could only ever be a short term ruse. Pretty soon they had an apartment in Rathmines and money was being left about the place. Clothes were being bought, sometimes strange, sexy clothes that Liam could not envisage on his country-girl woman who was then still a teenager of nineteen. He was thirty-seven; Linda always preferred older men. She told him that she was getting a hand-out from her own family; other times she would tell him she had a loan or that there had been money left to her by a relative in America and she was purchasing on the strength of its coming through. Of the late-night trips twice or three times a week, Linda always told Liam that she was visiting her sisters who lived in the greater Dublin area at the time. She knew from the outset that sooner or later she would have to tell him the truth if their relationship was to stand any chance of surviving: that she had become a prostitute. With her tall, sculpted features, her shock of natural blonde hair, and her non-threatening soft Border county accent, this beautiful – and young – new kid on the block was much in demand by the punters in search of paid sex.

Liam nearly lost his reason when she told him what her nocturnal travels were really all about. For a while he refused to believe it. Like so many women before her, she resolved that she would not remain at the game for a minute longer than it took to get her and Liam established, which at that point meant getting Liam's business up and running. But for Linda and Liam, like most of the rest of the world, life is what happens when you're busy making other plans. 'It just drifted on and on like so many other things in life and here I am nearly twenty years later,' Linda Lavelle says today.

After two months on the streets she got the flat in Rathmines, a teeming transient south city suburb given over to rented accommodation, and, in the early 1970s, the nearest thing Ireland had to a genuine cosmopolitan quarter with student flat dwellers of many nationalities, Jewish landlords and hoping-to-be-permanently-settled-soon country types like Linda and Liam and their baby son.

Within a few months she was off the streets and working in one of the many seedy little sex-rub joints that mushroomed in the city in the 1970s. Her resolve to extricate herself from sin soon weakened. There was huge money there for the taking in this game, she rationalised. And, compared to the paltry sum she had got as a waitress in a County Wexford hotel for all those long thankless hours with the prospects of waiting for ever to see Liam's business plans bear fruit, this was a doddle. Vice, she decided from a very early point in her apprenticeship, was nice. Very nice indeed. What's more, she was good at it and, yes, she did enjoy it – 'it' being what she describes today as her relationship with clients.

'I wouldn't ever have wanted to work at anything else once I started in this game. Every client is different and there's a great buzz out of meeting them and looking after them. No matter what happens to me in the future, I hope I can end my working days somehow connected to all of this. Psychologists and social commentators may have a view on this. It's about time we, the women they are getting paid to analyse publicly, had our say on prostitution and prostitutes . . . and our clients. A lot of us really do enjoy our work. We enjoy being professionals.

We're not a group of drug-addicted or alcoholic women who were raped by their fathers as kids and who are therefore emotionally flawed in some way. It doesn't work like that.'

It wasn't long before Linda Lavelle and her prostitute friend Jan Tyler opened up their own premises in Harold's Cross Road, a flatland suburb close to Rathmines but with a slightly more settled population. Her clients from her time on the streets followed her there; and on again from Harold's Cross Road to the love of her life . . . the Kasbah in the year of our Lord 1981. It was named with little appropriateness after the Kasbah Shopping Centre, a market mall in Gran Canaria in the Canary Islands where Linda Lavelle and her family still spend many of their holidays enjoying the fruits of her labours in the vineyards of Dublin's sin bins. 'There was something about the word "Kasbah" which seemed just right: it was full of Arabic mystery and sin!'

Six months after the terms of the lease had been agreed by Marion Murphy and with most of Linda's savings ploughed into renovating the basement of 60B, the doors on a new and unlikely to be surpassed era in sexual deviation in Ireland were about to be opened. New ceilings, floors, partitions, heating and plumbing systems were in place. (The external wooden stairwell was replaced with an iron one a few years later because of the opportunities it presented to passing pyromaniacs and sundry head cases.)

Liam was still there, long since recovered from the shock of being partnered to a woman who was, for some of their time at least, a woman who belonged to other men: strange men. His expertise in the construction business was invaluable to Linda. They had three children by this time and were living the life of suburban respectability in an up-market north city housing suburb where they live to this day.

Linda's plans for the Kasbah were always different. She had gone through her share of the bad days, 'the 1970s thing' as she calls it. She had been a part-time flat mate to Lyn Grey (nee Madden) for close on eight months in 1976/7 when they shared Lyn's flat in the south city suburb of Donnybrook and which Linda used as a base for carnal reward, dividing her time between there and her family's home in Rathmines. She knew first hand of Lyn's dreadful life and times at the hands of a psychopathically disturbed pimp called John Cullen who was eventually sent down for the murder of former prostitute Dolores Lynch, her mother Kathleen, and aunt Hannah. It was just another chapter in a decade of violence against the prostitutes at hands of rival pimp gangs from Dublin and Britain engaged in territorial wars on the lucrative streets of the capital.

Massage parlours – even the shoddy ones with a malevolent pimp in the background – offered the women more than they could ever hope for on streets, particularly in terms of physical comfort, personal safety, and a sense of being part of a collective. And for the first time in Ireland, these women's' clients were being offered sexual adventures that were simply impossible to engage in in the back of a car down a cul-de-sac off Fitzwilliam Square or the Pepper Canister church on Mount Street, with one eye cocked for a passing policeman or woman.

Something else was to happen in the early 1980s which had a profound effect on prostitution in Ireland. It was a decision by the highest judicial platform in the land, the Supreme Court, that made offences dealing with loitering or soliciting by a 'common prostitute' under the Vagrancy Act of 1898 inoperable under the terms of the 1937 Irish Constitution.

Up to that point the police normally attempted to prove that an accused woman was a 'common prostitute' by one of two ways. They adduced evidence that the woman had been found loitering or soliciting and warned by them on more than one occasion before that to which the charge before the court related. Alternatively, they adduced evidence of the accused's previous convictions for loitering or soliciting.

Effectively, these were crimes of condition or of character: a woman could be punished for prostitution merely on the basis of her reputation in the eyes of the police. The prosecution was not required to prove that the accused had engaged in any overt act in order to show criminal intent on her part.

In 1981, this procedure ran foul of the Supreme Court in the case of King vs The Attorney General – which struck down the creation of offences in over-broad terms such as the ones outlined.

Although drafted to target loiterers, Section 14 (11) of the Dublin Police Act 1842 was most often used by Irish police to give evidence that, in their opinion, the person in the dock was a prostitute – an opinion which, at the time, carried currency as evidence. Once the Supreme Court ruling was made, the lower courts took the view that evidence relating to the character of the defendant was only relevant to sentencing – that is, to the severity or otherwise of the penalty imposed *after* conviction.

The King decision was invoked by the defence in the case of Garda Kellegher vs Patricia Cullen and Others in the District Court under Section 4 (11) of the Dublin Police Act (1842) the year following the Supreme Court ruling. The basis of the decision was centred among other things on the use of the words 'common prostitute' as evidence of character before conviction.

The police were forced yet again to turn their attention to the statute books to enable them to secure convictions. This time it was Section 5 of the Summary Jurisdiction (Ireland) Amendment Act (1871). This empowered an officer who found a prostitute and/or her client coitally engaged to bring a charge under 'aiding and abetting indecent or criminal exposure'. But this, too, was a difficult law under which to obtain results in court as it allowed the accused to put up a defence of being an innocent courting couple, a tactic which proved almost impossible to argue successfully against under the ethos of 'beyond reasonable doubt' enshrined in Irish law.

The police had been rendered virtually impotent in their fight against both organised and one-off cases of prostitution as they turned to a rag bag of statutes such as the Town Improvement (Ireland) Act (1854) and the Town Police Clauses Act (1847) which dealt with 'common prostitutes' and 'night walkers' under various loitering-related offences.

Section 16 (1) of the Criminal Law Amendment Act (1935), provided that every 'common prostitute' who is found loitering in any street, thoroughfare, or other place, and importuning or soliciting passers-by for the purposes of prostitution or being otherwise offensive to passers-by shall be guilty of an offence. On conviction a woman was liable, in the case of a first offence, to a fine not exceeding £2 and in the case of a second offence to imprisonment for no longer than six months.

It is striking that key words in all these offences were not defined. The term 'common prostitute' fell to the courts for interpretation and they took the view that it covered a situation where a woman offered her body for sexual acts for payment, even where there was no sexual intercourse. 'Loitering' was not defined, either, but the courts took the view that it covered dawdling or lingering or travelling indolently on the public streets. It also, the courts decided, included loitering in a vehicle.

The view was held by the judicial system that loitering for prostitution was an offence even if a woman did not actively solicit customers – it was sufficient if she lingered with the intention that men should approach her. Soliciting required that a woman be physically present and that she engage in conduct involving gestures or acts to obtain prospective customers. A woman could solicit a prospective customer, therefore, from a window looking into a street. In such a case the offence of soliciting, from a legal point of view, took place on the street.

As with prostitution and soliciting, the police were forced to delve into the statute books of the last century and the early part of this one to deal with pimps and organised prostitution under the Criminal Law Amendment Act (1912) and the Vagrancy Act (1898).

The penalties for vice-related offences were risible and did not cause hardship to even the most financially hard pressed of the women. Convictions, however, could be catastrophic for them: the one abiding fear in the lives of most prostitutes is that those near and dear to them, sometimes mother and father, boyfriend, children, even husbands – would one day discover the lie under which they lived. A conviction carries with it a record which can be brought up almost without notice and if there is a Damocles Sword hanging over the heads of these women then this is surely it. This was another reason why the massage parlours were proving so popular with the street girls: vice-related summonses rarely found their way into the hands of the staff, or 'masseuses'.

Up to the Supreme Court ruling on evidence in 1981 there were 600 convictions for prostitution in Ireland; the number dropped by over one third the following year and after that it slumped to almost zero.

The drawing of the State prosecution's teeth allowed sex workers to carry out their business above ground, and made the introduction of sex dens or massage parlours infinitely more attractive than trudging the streets as bait for the passing kerb crawlers. It also enabled many prostitutes to break free from the clutches of underground pimps who, up to that point, had tried to justify themselves with the argument that they were protecting the women from the police and the rigours of the law. Interestingly, it also enabled prostitutes to avail themselves of health care when the need arose.

The old laws dealing with prostitution, soliciting and loi-tering were rightly consigned to the legal history section of the academic curriculum at the police training centres.

Instead, the police targeted the legal owners, landlords and

Madams who ran such brothels under 'keeping', 'knowing', and 'managing' charges brought under various Sections of the Criminal Law Amendment Act (1935), which was designed to deal with female prostitution only.

As a direct consequence of the Supreme Court ruling, safe sex was introduced into Ireland – at least it was legally safe for the first time for the vast majority of the prostitutes working in the massage parlours which numbered thirty-eight in Dublin in 1982. With the proliferation of the brothels, the vice girls had taken what no politician, no feminist agitator, no well-meaning liberal thinker, no women's interest group, and no trades union, ever succeeded in giving to them: that was acceptable working conditions largely of their own choice and a degree, at least, of immunity from the law.

It is ironic that in the summer of 1993, a Minister for Justice and one-time active women's rights sympathiser, Maire Geoghegan-Quinn, removed almost overnight those very conditions with a new set of formidable penalties introduced in the Criminal Law (Sexual Offences) Act (1993) aimed specifically at the massage parlours, the prostitutes and the clients.

The Act was intended to decriminalise gay sexual activity between consenting adults and to put it on an equal footing with heterosexual activity. Very little time was devoted in the Irish Parliament to debating that reform – most of the energies went instead on reshaping and extending the law on prostitution. It was as if Mrs Geoghegan-Quinn and her fellow legislators felt they had to adopt a moralistic approach to prostitution in case the public got the mistaken impression that they were adopting a liberal agenda by reforming the law on gay sexual activity. The Minister herself had long accepted that prostitution was a social problem yet here she was introducing heavy fines and terms of imprisonment for prostitutes and their clients, presenting the women as criminals in the eyes of the law.

Under pressure from a small but motivated group of

Opposition politicians, the Minister modified some of the punishments.

What Mrs Geoghegan-Quinn has succeeded in doing, apart from appeasing the right-wing moralist lobby within her own Fianna Fáil Party, is to put prostitution back in the same environment that led to so much injustice, hurt and violence that characterised it two decades earlier – 'the 1970s thing', as Linda Lavelle calls it. The new laws had hardly been in operation for a few days when the rot set in and squabbles broke out among the street girls and the women from the massage parlours who had gone back on the streets to make their living, rationalising perhaps wrongly that they were legally less vulnerable on the streets given the new legal climate. It is a scenario which will be repeated constantly as long as the current situation exists. And it is only a matter of time before the rival women turn to male protection to safeguard their patches and the pimps return on an organised and hideous level.

In April 1994 Marion Murphy lost her appeal against conviction for brothel-keeping at the Kasbah. The event was marked with a couple of paragraphs in the national newspapers. There was no such publicity for a legal event in the same week that took place in the Lower District Court where Tanya (not her real name) was appearing on similar charges relating to premises known as Rosebud in the city. A legal dispute over the serving of a search warrant stopped the case from going ahead, but not before a number of male witnesses had been called to give evidence. Linda Lavelle had implored Tanya to insist that the clients' full names be recorded in court instead of numbers and initials. And so it was. It would have been some consolation to Ms Murphy.

Four months earlier two women sat in my car as had been arranged the previous week. It was three o'clock on a freezing January morning on Dublin's Fitzwilliam Square. Across the road from us a youngish nun was dispensing biscuits and hot tea preserved in thermoses from the back of a van. Here, on the streets outside the nerve centre of the Irish medical world where Ireland's most eminent specialists hold their private clinics, the vice laws introduced the previous summer were already beginning to bite deep into the psyche of the prostitutes.

One of the women pointed to her swollen eye and spoke of the client who gave it to her. 'I was looking after a client – he was an oral client. Suddenly he had his hands around my mouth and throat. I felt my eyes were bulging. I fell to the ground and he started kicking my face in. He burst my lips and did this to my eye. But that's okay in a way: you stand out there [on the streets] and you expect some trouble now and again from the clients and sometimes from the other girls. It doesn't happen all that often. It's not easy money but you stand out there. I was out there the other night from ten o'clock until three in the morning . . . out there in the cold and the rain and the fear and I made £80. Five hours work and I made eighty fucking miserable pounds. But that's okay, too. There's nights like that and you have to put up with it.'

Her sister in prostitution nodded in agreement.

Both women have been selling their sex on the streets for over a decade. When Linda Lavelle describes such women as street girls she serves to underline two distinct classes within Irish vice. For the women who sat with me in the car that night seemed to have few life skills and clearly appeared to me as women under enormous oppression. Thinking of them as criminals as the law categorises them is simply an outrageous violation of truth. For them, the new vice laws have made their existence more wretched and more precarious than ever. Almost every night they are being visited by policemen and women warning them to move on or face prosecution. The pimps – the kind who patrolled the streets, menacing and exploiting women in the 1970s – are back out in force feeding off the increased number of women who have been forced out of the massage parlours and onto the streets by the new legislation They are not safe here, either.

'We've got offers from pimps,' one of them told me. 'You know, protection offers. It's only a matter of time before we have to join them and pay them money to protect us. We know it's a rip-off because we're only paying them to protect us from them. But there's too many girls out here now and you need to have someone who you're paying to protect your interests against the girls who are not paying anyone and who are cluttering up the streets and taking all the business.'

This second woman who was in a state of distress for most of our encounter said simply, 'I will not get off the street until I get a job. God, I'm 33 years of age and by this time I should have a husband and some children and I've nothing. I have five babies by five different fathers. I have been kicked around the streets while I was still pregnant. Now I can't have a baby even though I'm trying. The new legislation isn't going to stop anything – it has just made things worse for everyone, including the people who are not prostitutes or their clients but who are coming home from a dance or a disco and who can now be stopped by the police for loitering. I have seen that happen, you know.'

She added, 'And what about the rapists and the muggers and all the people with problems who came to prostitutes on the street before? Do you honestly think that they are going to stop?'

Neither woman was impressed by the deterrents in the new laws. The freedom to choose an alternative way of making a living is one they say they do not have, and now they languish in the further ignominy of being classed as common criminals.

Such lofty matters of jurisprudence and institutionalised injustice, however, would have been far from the mind of the attractive housewife as she prepared school lunches for her three young children on the morning of 20 May 1981. She had a business to run and today was the grand opening of a place which would preoccupy her life for the next decade and with which she would very soon become synonymous and, arguably, emotionally bonded to. 'I totally adored the Kasbah. I felt totally, totally at home there. It meant more to me than my own home. They were the happiest days of my life.'

The Kasbah's days and nights had begun and hedonism in Ireland had arrived on a stupendous scale.

Chapter Five

'We Were Total Whores'

Mandy and Charlene looked up in disbelief at the gum-chewing apparition that had just floated in through the front door dressed in a red leather mini-skirt and black fishnet tights, with her pouting red lips locked on a cigarette, her straight jet-black shoulder length hair, wet and brushed back.

Mandy Jameson broke the silence, whether or not breakage was required. 'My Jesus, Linda, if you were looking for tarts, total and utter fucking tarts, then you've got one this time. You're in the tarts business big time now, girl. You're going all the fucking way.'

Linda Lavelle remembered looking up from the omnipresent blazing coal fire and not bothering to respond to Mandy's predictable invective. New girls received a baptism of fire in the Kasbah and places like it and, she thought, there was no reason to shield this one from it. Charlene, who looked more motherly and middle class than Mandy (although she was neither) offered the new girl, who called herself Vikki, her hand.

'Don't mind her, love,' she said, looking towards Mandy. 'She was born to be a lady but there weren't any vacancies at the time and she never got over it.'

Vikki couldn't have known it at the time but she and Mandy had something in common: they had both told me that at that point in their careers they enjoyed sex. ('Course I do. There's girls'll tell you that they don't but they're just trying to fool you into thinking they're some sort of martyrs. Don't fucking mind them, Dave. Course they like it.' Vikki had spoken these words to me whenever that well-worn but still intriguing topic of prostitutes, sex and the question of enjoyment arose.)

And as time went on, Mandy and Vikki would share other things, too, like a high-ranking Catholic churchman, among their legions of paid lovers. (Mandy often boasted that she was okay for the Hereafter, having two such clerical dignitaries sipping from the trough of her carnal delights.)

Vikki genuinely didn't much mind the 'apparition' jibe. She came from the school of hard knocks in north inner-city Dublin, although this was her inauguration into the world of hired vice. Anyway, she had inured herself to whatever sensitivities she might have had that day with a few cannabis joints – a habit which was to become her calling card.

Linda eyed up her new girl. 'You know what sort of place this is, Vikki? You know what sort of job we do in a place like this?'

'Ah, yeah,' came Vikki's reply, her young voice was already crackling from too many cigarettes. 'It's a brothel. That's why I'm here, Linda.' Linda had good feelings about this Dublin woman in her early twenties who had all the mannerisms and the appearance of a female version of Keith Richards. While good looks counted, they were only ever in second place to guile and this new girl seemed to have plenty of that.

Linda's assessments in relation to brothel management always seemed to me to be both immaculate and thorough. 'You could have Kim Bassinger in here in the morning and it wouldn't make a bit of difference if she doesn't have attitude. Men like to feel that you are glad to see them, even though they know you're doing it for money, for their money. Many clients would say: "What can I do for you" and if a girl replies, "No, no, I'm, here to give you pleasure" then that's got to be a turn-off for the client . . . it's the ice cold Madam job. Girls have got to be able to say to their client, "You have to please me."'

She was to be proved right about Vikki. Too right, perhaps. 'Vikki ended up making perverts more perverted! She really loved her business and would often leave a room with her hair matted to her head in perspiration she'd get into the work so much.'

Vikki started work there and then, taking her place on the red, grey and black sofa along with Charlene and Mandy who were using words she could only remember from her short-lived school days and that, applied in this place, confused her. Words like Discipline, Correction, Frustration, Head-mistresses and Schoolgirls' Uniforms. They were used mostly as adjectives and very often in the context of the strangely theatrical term, Madhatters' Night. It was her first encounter with what the Kasbah was really all about and much, much later, when asked what made the Kasbah so different, she told me, 'Some of the girls working in the other parlours [brothels] wear those white coats and shoes and have themselves convinced that they're some kind of fucking sex therapists. But I'll tell you, Dave, they're screwing and fucking and sucking every man that comes into the place. It was never like that in the Kasbah: none of that oul white coats shite. In the Kasbah we were total whores. Total whores.'

Beyond the sofa and on the other side of the bottle-green curtain a businessman client was asking Linda about the availability of new girls. Young Vikki's time had come.

'All the rooms were engaged at the time,' recalled Linda. 'And quick as a flash Vikki asked whether there was any room out in the back. And Vikki meant any room, as opposed to any rooms. That was her style.'

She took her middle-aged client through the hallway to the coal house outside, agreed terms and firmly planted her feet on two pots of gloss paint to avoid getting her red patent shoes dirty and, hey presto, 'I gave that nice man the best bit of doggy he'd ever had,' said Vikki later. 'He left the place on

Cloud Nine. I bet he was never whored in a coal house before!'

If Vikki was a rough-hewn Dubliner, Mandy on the other hand, was the archetypal redheaded Irish convent-educated girl from the sticks. She was known to neighbours and friends as well behaved and mannerly in the town in the southern half of Ireland where she grew up – a good girl. She was born to well-to-do parents who, while strict in their application of the Roman Catholic ethos within the family, doted on their daughter. Mandy was what the psychologists refer to as the 'hero child'.

She fulfilled both her own and her parents' middle-class expectations in every respect and when she married a local businessman and leading light in the nearby town's Chamber of Commerce, life went on autopilot: destination dull, predictable respectability, the contented mother in a bungalow on half-an-acre of land just outside town. Her social credentials were further enhanced by that uniquely Irish status symbol of having relations in the cloth. She had two cousins in the priesthood, another three were nuns. There was a time after she finished college in the mid-1970s when she considered becoming a Bride of Christ herself. The nearest she came to it, however, was in sacrificing her body on the altar of lust for a powerful member of the Catholic clergy who to this day uses Mandy and other prostitutes who were once part of the Kasbah scene. (Not surprisingly, Vikki was another one of his favourites. He shared her penchant for the 'wacky baccy' – cannabis cigarettes – which she brought in ample supply for all-night sex sessions in a top Dublin hotel. The churchman would always arrive with a male companion and hire two of the girls who would come around to the hotel for a night of sex and smoking.)

Mandy's marriage didn't work out, despite having three children. Physical and verbal abuse became the norm in her union with Sam (not his real name). He regularly (and inaccurately at the time) taunted her with being a prostitute, something which tests her middle-class conscience to this day.

She ended up stabbing him several times in the chest after one of their many blazing rows. (He was held in intensive care for several days after losing four pints of blood.) She eventually left him and, like so many girls who find themselves in the vice business, first got a job in catering – in a restaurant in a nearby town. For one year she kept things going for herself and her two young boys and their little sister. When the eatery folded, Mandy joined the caravan of young people in Ireland at the time who were looking towards the big cities at home and beyond for their salvation.

She spent the first six months in Dublin in a women's refuge where she befriended a young Belfast woman called Beverly (not her real name), another escapee from a failed relationship. The two women eventually found a flat for themselves on Dublin's northside, thanks to an uncle of Mandy's who had shown her occasional but genuine kindness. After collecting their dole money every Thursday they would make their way to the Wind Jammer, an early morning docklands pub, where they would commiserate with one another for several hours at a time. One morning, a small, fat man sidled up to Beverly who was then eighteen years old. 'What's wrong? You pair look very low in yourselves altogether. Are ye looking for work?' Beverly spilled out her tale of woe and self-pity. Mandy was intensely shy of men at that point in her life and as usual she was content to let her companion do the confessing for both of them. (Much later she told me, 'I was not wised up to men at all when I arrived in Dublin. My husband was the only man I really even spoke to. When I started at the Kasbah the first question I asked Linda was whether I take my clothes off right away or wait until the man tells me to.')

The Fat Man promised Beverly that he could secure gainful employment for her. No hitches. No strings. The following day she was in the Kasbah, much to the incredulity and disapproval of Mandy. 'You can't do this,' she told her when she arrived home from her first day's work as a prostitute. 'We'll get by somehow without this. You know you're a prostitute, Beverly? You're a whore and no whore is sleeping with my kids, you fucking tramp.'

Two shifts at the Kasbah later had changed attitudes dramatically. Seemingly impervious to criticism and character assassination, Beverly continued to regale Mandy with stories of easy money and a barrel of laughs in her new found employment. 'You should have seen the money she was making for a few hours work,' Mandy told me. 'She split her sides telling me about the £150 she raked in off of a little fella they all called Chinese Sammy for a fucking hour and a half's work.'

That afternoon Mandy was down in the Kasbah talking with Linda Lavelle about the hardships of life on the dole for a still youngish twenty-seven-year-old mother. Linda listened like a sister confessor. She had become used to 'new women' exercising the need to rationalise and possibly deny their feelings of guilt at what they were contemplating. Mandy confided to Linda that she had a boyfriend but he was not much use on the financial front, she said, although he did provide food. Linda's response was, as usual, direct without being offensively so. 'You're better off in here riding for money than being at home every night riding for rashers, Mandy.'

She was told to come back at five that evening for the night shift. Mandy's day was spent taking one of her little sons to Our Lady's Hospital for Sick Children in the southside suburb of Crumlin. He had developed a severe chest infection. She had to walk home from the city centre on the final leg of her four-bus journey when the money ran out. Money was always running out. Mandy resolved that this was no way to live: she had done the right thing by meeting Linda and agreeing to work in the Kasbah and the long walk home was the vindication she needed to fortify her for teatime at the Kasbah in a black mini-skirt which had seen much better days.

Some years later Mandy would meet her husband quite by

accident in O'Connell Street, Dublin's main thoroughfare. The encounter freed the anger she had long managed to hold down thanks to a well established relationship with vodka and white lemonade. 'Hi, Sam. Do you remember me? I'm your wife, Sam. Do you remember calling me a prostitute and a whore, Sam? Well have I got news for you. *I am* a fucking prostitute now thanks to fucking you. And the men I have now treat me a damn sight better than you ever did, you fucking bastard.'

The nonplussed man put his hands to his face and started crying uncontrollably in the middle of the crowded street. Mandy Jameson walked away with an outward swagger of conquest.

She was always too clever, too defensive, and perhaps too resentful, to allow me near the source of her inner turmoil which manifested itself in a constant state of being angry with people and things whenever we met.

Charlene Robertson's introduction to the life of 'hotel businesswoman' (as she likes to refer to her 'escorting' pastimes) and sometime masseuse at the Kasbah Health and Fitness Studio on Mountjoy Square, came at the relatively advanced age of thirty-five. Like Mandy, it too, had a religious flavour to it when one of the first people to learn of her fall from grace was the Vatican's Papal Nuncio to Ireland, Monsignor Dr Gaetano Alibrandi. She had made an appointment to see the venerable churchman, then the Pope's official emissary to Ireland and a man who had justifiably earned a reputation for upholding the Catholic Church's unflinching stand on matters of faith and morality, at his opulent residence at the Phoenix Park. The seeing of couples whose marriages had run into difficulties was one of the many good works of the churchman's mission rarely visible to the public. Charlene had agreed to see him in response to her husband's efforts to have the marriage annulled by the Church. ('I'm going to tell the bishops of Ireland all about that two-faced bollocks,' she told friends at the time.)

In a matter-of-fact kind of way, the homely blonde told the austere looking but mild-mannered Sicilian cleric that she was a prostitute. 'What's more, your worship, my husband was my very first client. He was the first man ever to pay me for sex.' Charlene wasn't joking. She revealed to the bemused churchman how the two of them hadn't had 'it' for years and that, one night, he became so desperate for sex that he offered her £20 for intercourse. 'I agreed and told him to leave the money on the dresser where I could see it before he got into bed,' she told the attentive churchman. Come Friday of the same week, Charlene noticed that she was £20 short of her housekeeping allowance. Her husband told her that he had given her the balance earlier that week in the bedroom. He could distinctly remember leaving a £20 note on the dresser by the bed. 'And what's more, your worship' – Charlene was warming to her task in front of the Nuncio who remained inscrutable throughout, 'he's the only man I've ever had who took the money back after he got what he wanted. How's that for a swine?' The grand old churchman shook her hand and showed her to the door. 'Nisameetinga you, youla be hearing soona. Guudbio.'

As I envisaged these three women, more disparate than desperate, thrown together by fate and sitting together on the striped sofa in the Kasbah that day with the exotic names God had, perhaps, never intended for them, I couldn't help thinking how close they were in many ways to women I knew elsewhere. Mandy and Charlene could be my neighbours, they could be the babysitters or the mother who telephones the newspaper where I work complaining about the high cost of school books. Was it solely personal circumstance that put these women here? Or was there an aberration, an emotional, spiritual or moral fault line that I could not see that had brought them here to this part of Dublin once fondly known as Monto.

This had been the first moral battleground of the Legion of Mary and its inspired leader Frank Duff who succeeded in ridding the area of prostitutes, hotels of ill repute and the low-life criminals who managed them when it was the only police no-go area in Europe. That was in the 1920s when Monto's infamy was recognised in the tenth edition of *Encyclopaedia Britannica* thus: 'Dublin seems to form an exception to the usual practice in the United Kingdom. In that city the police permit open brothels confined to one area, but carried on more openly than in the south of Europe or even Algiers.'

It was estimated that as many as 200 prostitutes operated openly in the area during that time.

But Duff and loyal acolytes could not have envisaged this Ireland – this Monto – of the 1980s and 1990s. The women he had to rescue from moral depravity were not difficult to identify as victims of a patriarchal society. Nor was it difficult to identify the men pimps and the clients and the usually ruthless Madams of the time, so unlike their counterparts of modern Ireland. In the Kasbah on that dry June afternoon in 1982, it was so different, so unclear when it came to knowing who to forgive, who to blame, and who to feel sad for as the deep warm Continental voice filtered through the bottle-green velvet curtain . . .

'Ello, Linda. My Mistress Linda. 'Ow are you today, my dearest? I've got the money outside in my briefcase. Shall I tell Gert to bring it in?'

The curtain swished back. 'Girls,' said Linda standing hand-in-hand with this tall dark stranger in his mid-forties wearing the tailor-made Gucci suit, 'I would like you to meet Lauden [not his real name]. Lauden, this is Vikki, Mandy and Charlene.' I remember feeling disconcerted yet intrigued as Linda retold this episode. She gave me the impression that she and Lauden had looked as starry-eyed as a couple of teenagers about to head off on their first date together. She was, of course, putting on another Oscar-winning performance for Lauden, one of the Kasbah's many clients who risked everything for these strange, ethereal hours. For Lauden was a high-ranking diplomat who had been attached to an embassy in Ireland for the past two years. Earlier that same day Linda had given him £1,000 to convert into pesetas for her forthcoming holiday to the Canaries. She always got the embassy rate from Lauden. She also charged him something of an embassy rate for her services, a kind of each-way winner was Lauden.

As a senior member of a heavyweight diplomatic mission in Ireland, he didn't raise any eyebrows in the office when he put in for such sums. None of his colleagues could have dreamt that Lauden, as well as being a career diplomat, was also a Slave who derived his pleasures from unquestioning sub-servience to the woman he always called Mistress Linda: as a Slave she was his boss and he would do anything she told him to do. That was his fantasy. And when Linda went off on holiday he would take leave from the embassy when he could and stay at the Kasbah day and night, doing the laundry, hoovering the carpets, getting the fire lit in the mornings and making sure that Linda's 'book money' was being properly put aside for payment into the bank every afternoon. Vikki recalled the day when Lauden came back from the laundrette with towels and linen while Linda was sunning herself on a Gran Canarian beach. 'He went fucking crazy when he realised that he'd left Linda's bag – a fifty pence fucking plastic bag – in the laundrette. He ran back down the street shrieking, "I must get Linda's bag. Linda's bag, I must get it back. Oh no, oh no."'

The Man From The Embassy was also deeply possessive of Linda. He always insisted on driving her to the airport and even went to the trouble of checking with the tour operator exactly when her flight was due back. Once he sped out to Dublin Airport in his chauffeur-driven limo to receive and at the same time check up on his beloved Mistress Linda. 'He was insanely jealous and had to satisfy himself that I wasn't going away with a man.' She was, of course, going off with her long-time companion Liam and she had a job convincing Lauden that the man standing by her side and looking fit and tanned was really her older brother.

Some time later Lauden was officiating at a diplomatic fixture on board a warship berthed in Dublin Port for a few days and which was open to public viewing: exchanging niceties and glad handing it with a couple of political nondescripts from City Hall on special municipal invitation was all part and parcel of his calling and he did it reluctantly but with his usual aplomb. When he saw the handsome brother of Linda Lavelle make his way up the gangplank with three children he recognised as hers (he had met them in the Kasbah on several occasions) he mused to himself just how small – and potentially dangerous – a place like Dublin could be. He was just about to reintroduce himself to the man he had met in the airport and who had taken such good care of his woman when one of the children shrieked: 'Daddy, daddy, please can we see the big gun now? Please!'

Lauden was not a man to show his emotions, at least not while on duty. He smoothly reached into a jacket pocket and took out an instamatic camera before reintroducing himself to Linda's 'brother' with a firm but courteous handshake.

A week later he was giving Linda one of her many lifts home in the big black limo with the bullet-proof glass. This time, however, the bullets were going off inside the car.

'You never told me you had a husband.' He managed to look conversationally impassive, recalled Linda, as he stared through the heavily tinted window away from her.

'I don't. I don't, Lauden. Who's been telling you lies?' Linda was, as usual, putting on an Oscar-winning scene: it was never deceit, never something personal to her, just old-fashioned professionalism. It was business.

This time she was spiked, however. Lauden had the photographic evidence in his wallet and he produced it with a kind of studied anger. It would have been little comfort to either of them that up to that point she was, technically at least, telling the truth because she was, in fact, single.

'Who in fuck's name is this then, your brother? And why in fuck's name were your kids calling him "daddy"?' His mellow accent was now a victim to rage and betrayal as he stamped his index finger almost right through the snapshot.

'Fuck you!'

Linda was mildly concerned for her safety: that was all. Deception was something she was paid to do. The fact that this time reality got in the way and spoiled things for Lauden was his tough shit, not hers.

After Lauden realised that Linda was no longer *his* woman and never had been, he continued to attend the Kasbah for straight sex (for him that meant lying down naked on the flat of his back and having the girl do all the work. He never once changed his preferences) rather than fantasy. He completely ignored her, turning his attentions to other girls including Lis O'Brien (not her real name), Charlene, Mandy, and a girl I'll call Louise. There were no more cheap pesetas.

(Linda and the other girls didn't have to wait very long for a return of favourable conditions on the international money market, however: a senior figure in the Irish tourism industry whom they had christened Dollars George (George was not his real Christian name) saw to that. He would always pay the girls in US dollars but could be prevailed upon to settle his bill in other currencies if asked nicely to do so.)

Lauden had no more gifts for Linda. No more lifts home in the dead of night in the bullet-proof limousine. No more Happy Christmas cards. No more sweet talk of his 'Mistress Linda'. But Lauden didn't try and make Linda jealous, as some suitors might have. 'I think he was scared that if he tried that I would have barred him, and he never wanted that to happen,' Linda told me. 'Sure I didn't give a shit.'

Lauden has since left Ireland for another diplomatic posting.

Chapter Six

Dire Straits To El Dorado

Street-wise members of the Irish police force had learned to live with, metaphorically of course, the bordellos and the prostitutes who worked in them long before the Kasbah opened its doors in 1981. At worst it was an ambivalent relationship: the law was being flouted, sometimes overtly, at many of the parlours. They were also opening at a rate of knots in the early 1980s as the ramifications of the King appeal in the Supreme Court (see p.50) led many prostitutes to believe that they had gone an inch beyond the reach of the law. But it was their very success, upturning the old cliché about safety in numbers, which ensured that some action would have to be taken sooner or later if the police were not to become seriously embarrassed.

On the other hand, the bordellos were never seen as either the source of or the reason for serious crime, and police action on vice operations remained low on their list of priorities. And there was always the added advantage to the police that some of the girls were willing to impart 'pillow talk' intelligence from some of their criminally orientated clients and their male friends and associates in return for minimum police attention. It was all infinitely more preferable to what had gone on in the city in the 1970s when Dublin's growing population of prostitutes literally took their lives in their hands each time they went out on the streets.

In the mid- and late 1970s, and unbeknown to the average Dubliner, a bloody territorial war was raging in the traditional red-light districts of Fitzwilliam Square, Baggot Street and the Pepper Canister church area. The charge was being directed, not from within, but from Derby in England by a Jamaican pimp gang led by the notorious Tyrone Fletcher who regularly flew scores of black prostitutes into Dublin backed up by heavy black muscle. The black women proved an instant success with their Irish clients who to that point would have had little or no opportunity to encounter people not of their own colour. At one point Fletcher's girls were sending his syndicate £3,000 a week home from Ireland. When a black-hating fellow Englishman called Johnny Grey, husband of the tragic figure of Cork-born prostitute Lyn Grey (see pp.48–9), confronted the Derby syndicate on the streets of Dublin all hell broke loose and the police hadn't the first idea how to handle it. They couldn't be faulted: up to that point the tell-tale signs of organised vice on such a scale had not existed in Ireland since the start of the century. Now, for no apparent reason, pitched street battles involving the pimps, their imported women and the highly aggrieved local girls were commonplace at night.

Detectives even asked Grey to inveigle the Derby-based gang and its leader, Mr Fletcher, to Dublin and they would take it from there. That never happened. Eventually they acceded to Grey's requests to handle it his own way, with the predictable caveat that he was not to break the law in the process. It was an unusual but appropriate stratagem for them to adopt: Grey was a pimp himself and had intimate knowledge of the Derby-based gang. It takes a thief . . .

But the real break for the police came when the *Sunday World* newspaper handed over a complete dossier on Dublin's major vice operations and the people behind them to the Director of Public Prosecutions. It was the spark that lit the fire under the vice business: the red-light areas looked more like scenes from prohibition Boston than peaceful, conservative

Ireland, as van loads of cops descended on the streetwalkers while uniformed police harassed their kerb crawling customers with drink-driving tests and the like. There was a huge increase in the number of vice girls charged, and a similar increase in the number of women who were prepared to snitch on their pimps, figuring that in this new dangerous and fractious climate they had just as much to fear from their male controllers as they had from the police.

Dublin was being cleaned up – not this time by the Legion of Mary – but by a racist pimp called Johnny Grey, the Irish police force and a newspaper team dedicated to, but rarely credited with, the campaigning side of its journalism.

Linda Lavelle had lived through it all, sharing a flat with Lyn Grey, later to become more widely known as Lyn Madden. She was on friendly terms with prostitute Dolores Lynch who perished in an inferno at her home along with her mother Kathleen and her aunt Hannah Hearne after one of the most ruthless men in Dublin, pimp John Cullen, had shoved fire lighters into her home in Hammon Street, sixteen days into 1983. Lyn Grey had been long-time lover of and worker for Cullen. It was no secret to either her or Linda Lavelle that Dolores Lynch – a reformed vice girl who had become a dedicated spokeswoman for prostitutes in Ireland – was high on his hit-list. Ms Lynch had given up the game in the late 1970s and began blowing the whistle on the pimps. She was one of the main contributors to a report on prostitution being drawn up at the time by Irish parliamentarian Michael Keating.

It was out of this furnace of mayhem and danger, of women bottle-slashed at the hands of a hundred Johnny Greys; of imported black musclemen beating her friend Lyn to a pulp; of wretched women, desperate mothers going into a game as a last refuge from poverty, that Linda Lavelle's instincts were forged. She had the intelligence and cunning and survival instincts to create something lasting out of the emergence of the sex-rub shops. A new El Dorado of vice was just waiting to be discovered, this time by a woman, and that fact more than any other was to become hugely significant for the prostitutes of Dublin for over a decade.

Until the early 1990s Linda Lavelle had little cause for concern when it came to formal police interest in her affairs. The bad old days were over and the parlours' Madams would only receive untoward police attention if they were either stupid or sloppy and indiscreet. Linda was neither. (She would later take much professional pride in the fact that not a single condom was found during the raid on the Kasbah which led to the February 1993 brothel-keeping trial of Marion Murphy. They were all thrown into the fire.) Linda actually cultivated the visits of off-duty officers to the Kasbah who were engaged in the pursuit of valuable information more likely to be given on such 'unofficial' occasions when the tea, cigarettes and small talk replaced the slim black 'Garda' notebooks and pens. She made sure that girls under eighteen never worked for her. She had a reputation for spotting trouble a mile off, although she admits that that ability must have been out to lunch the day she took on Margaret 'Poppy' Healy as her co-manageress. Her girls were instructed to 'look after' policemen clients well and she even overlooked 'the book' – her £15 cut from every client – for some cop clients. Despite considerable lore to the contrary, I never discovered any evidence that the police force – the Garda Síochána – had an unduly high number of its men availing of the services of the massage parlour girls. 'We got on very well with the police,' recalled Linda. 'It was all very civilised. I remember when one drunken [County] Meath Gaelic football supporter crapped all over the towels in the shower and we called the cops. We thought he was going to get really nasty. Two uniformed officers arrived and one of them hauled this little bastard back into the shower and stood over him saying, "Do you expect these women to clean up the shit after you? Clean up your own shit." He then hauled him back out to – I think it was Ann – and said, "Did you pay that lady for her services? Now pay up and get out.'"

But there was one southside detective who had long since joined the ranks of what the girls describe as 'specialist' clients. It was far from tea and sympathy that brought the man they simply called The Policeman to the Kasbah. Maybe he explained to his wife that the weals on the backs of both his legs were sustained in the course of cornering a violent criminal – at the same time and location every fortnight: for he was a Discipline client who willingly submitted to having his flesh pummelled to pulp by a big lady called Maggie until he ejaculated.

Like virtually all clients of this peculiar form of masochism, standard forms of sexual activity didn't enter the frame: they were Slaves of a kind, men who felt so inferior, so beholden and so in awe of the woman who flailed them with a bamboo cane, that they would never deign to look for any form of sexual stimulation from them other than a beating. Charlene Robertson once told me, 'They wouldn't feel fit to kiss your feet on the way out the door. The Slaves just felt so grateful that they could get their punishment. The Policeman would leave the place with the blood dripping between the cheeks of his arse and down both legs. He left the place a very happy man.'

Linda Lavelle had experienced her first police raid back in 1980. It was a busy weekend in April. She was still a year away from taking charge of the Kasbah and was operating her vice base out of a house on Harold's Cross Road with her long time friend and fellow prostitute, Jan Tyler. They had taken on the services of another masseuse, Karla (not her real name), for the night, to cope with the demand of an explicably busy period.

It was unguarded horror that swept over the three women as two of their politician clients – Parliamentary members of the Fianna Fáil Party, Ireland's largest political grouping – were on the premises when the batons started hitting the locked wooden front door. The politicians, drinking buddies, had been in the house two nights before when they had hand-picked Linda and Karla for business the following night before

heading off to a political conference in the city centre to
address the decline in the fabric of Irish life. Linda recalls, 'All
the windows came in. Glass was shattered everywhere. One of
the TDs [the Irish equivalent of MP] was holding my hand
and saying how lovely I looked. I was wearing a see-through
blouse, that's all, and he was bollock-naked with a big horn on
him. When we heard the banging on the door we thought it
was gangsters. I remember being so relieved when they
shouted "It's the police, open up immediately."'

The other TD was in a partitioned bedroom, unaware of
what was going on out front and hardly reflecting on his
speech the previous night as he attempted to enhance the fabric of his own social life for all he was worth on top of a naked
and quite breathless Karla.

What happened next would have pleased the strong macho
element within the party founded by Eamon de Valera and
whose members proudly proclaimed themselves The Soldiers
of Destiny. For the TD holding his hand-picked prostitute's
hand in the front room didn't bat an eyelid as the ten cops
piled into the room, Linda recalled. He merely looked down as
if to check on the state of his manhood. When he found that
it was still erect he folded his arms in front of him, much like
Yul Brynner in *The King And I*, masking his own view of his
manhood. He proudly stood there in his pelt with a smile on
his face, still beside Linda, as the young female officer in a duf-
fle coat took down his particulars. Names were taken, the
usual legal warning issued. 'Anything you say may be taken
down and used in evidence . . .' Nothing ever came of the
1980 raid on the house in Harold's Cross. Not in a legal sense,
at any rate. The two politicians are still clients of Linda
Lavelle's, having out-lived both Harold's Cross Road and the
decade of decadence that was the Kasbah.

The raid itself proved a huge personal challenge to Linda
Lavelle's sense of judgement. 'I felt very secure at that time,
very safe with the police because we weren't causing bother

and they had never given any warnings, any indication, that something like this was going to happen. We got on really well with the police.'

The move to the Kasbah saw the reestablishment of good relations with the police: so much so that Linda wasn't adverse to calling on their services when the need arose, such as the time she feared that she was going to be 'rolled' by two gangster types who were inside 60B as clients. Two plainclothes officers arrived – one of them a young detective called Kevin Fields who would feature so centrally in the huge surveillance operation and raid on the Kasbah in September 1991 and the subsequent court case. 'I made the stupid mistake of thinking that officer Fields and the other officer were part of the same gang so I called the police station again and told them to hurry because other members of the gang had arrived!' said Linda. 'They sent up two uniformed officers and that's when I realised who Kevin Fields was. He was really very pleasant and good at his job.'

Apart from the politicians, three other household names were clients of the Kasbah back in the early months of its inception. They included two members of the judiciary (one insisted on being whipped while wearing fishnet tights and high-heeled shoes) and the politician who cleverly held his cool so as to ensure that he would not feature in the Central Criminal Court Case a decade later against Marion Murphy and the Kasbah, despite being recorded on video surveillance.

A good day at the Kasbah would see as many as forty clients pass through the door. The hoped-for El Dorado for Linda and her girls had arrived. (The record for one day was forty-eight.) Linda Lavelle put the average at twenty every day, seven days a week. One prostitute, Pia Masterson who was there almost from the start, described her earnings as colossal. 'I had a brilliant standard of living because of the Kasbah. Brilliant. There were days when I'd clear well over £800. You always figured your money by the day. Everything – clients, money, cops, was by the day. I remember one time being in a queue with some mothers in a supermarket and they were moaning on about their phone bills for £30 and £40 and wondering where they'd get the money to pay them. It was nothing unusual for me to get £400 bill and there was never any problem in paying it. I remember one Monday morning going into the Kasbah to start my shift. I was broke because we all lived up to the money we earned with new cars and good clothes and the likes. By Friday afternoon I had bought two tickets for a fortnight for two in Spain and I had £2,000 spending money as well. And it was like that every week.' When asked what were the busiest years, Linda Lavelle replied, 'We had ten years, ten peak years. It was busy all of the time. Even after we closed it stayed busy with the phone hopping all the time and clients still coming down the steps looking for business.'

In fact, the Kasbah opened twice after it was closed 'for good' in October 1991. By mid-December the doors were flung open for the season of goodwill, a gesture of eccentricity by Linda rather than a wreckless defiance of further interference from the police: it proved as sinful and as popular as ever and ensured a bountiful Christmas for the girls and, presumably, a more exciting one for the clients. In March of the following year Linda and Pia descended the steps once more, this time at the behest of Linda's partner Liam, who wanted the girls to retrieve some of the expensive fittings and fixtures they had installed over the years. Within the space of three-quarters of an hour, the two women had looked after four clients who just happened to call. Said Pia, 'It was as if things never changed . . . as if we had never closed in the first place. These four men had just come down on the off chance that the place would be open. And the phone was ringing all the time, too, but we didn't bother to answer.' Liam's expectations of collateral were not realised, but he could have comforted himself that both girls came back with their bank balances improved.

Earning power always owed more to expertise than looks, despite the misconception that the good-looking girls always got the clients while the 'dogs' were left with the scraps. The other facility for earning money depended on just how far a prostitute was prepared to go with the men referred to as the specialist clients; how deviant and perverse she was prepared to be. Pia was into full sex but not much more; other girls such as Vikki O'Toole, and later Margaret Healy, made large sums of money from engaging in the most lurid encounters with their clients. Yet Pia was making as much as any of them. 'I was a good listener and I gave good advice. And I had a knack for spotting a client with easy money and I made him feel very welcome, very loved. That's the art of the game, it's all fantasy. I would sit and listen to a client for ages about wife troubles or woman troubles or kid troubles or work troubles and I would be appreciated a lot for it.'

By 1983 the Kasbah was well into its halcyon era – an era which would last with few interruptions until 1991. It opened at 10.30am every day and closed at 10.30pm or 11pm seven days a week. There would rarely be more than four girls on any one of the daily two-shift system. It was not unusual for 140 clients to pass through the steel door and into the sins of the basement every week, although 120 was nearer the average. By now the Kasbah's reputation for welcoming 'every fucking possible type of looper', as Linda once called her more deviantly wayward clients, was firmly established.

One man from those early days was the politician whose disposition to illicit vice would become such an open secret eight years later in both political and journalistic circles.

Not until now could the story of his and other men's darkest secrets be told by the women who shared them.

Chapter Seven

The Schoolboy's Secrets

Like so many of his fellow travellers into the deviant world of illicit sexual pleasure, the Fine Gael politician who featured in the police video footage made during investigations leading to the Kasbah trial of 1993 seemed at stages quite uncaring of the enormous risks to which he was submitting himself, along with others close to him, during his frequent dangerous liaisons with the ladies of the bordello. In the early summer of 1991 many of the Kasbah's more regular and well connected clients had received unofficial and well intentioned warnings from the police that a raid was imminent. Several of them acted on that advice and stayed in the trenches until the surveillance operation had run its course. Others used Linda Lavelle's mobile phone service to set up appointments outside the pan of the video cameras operating in Mountjoy Square West and, as some correctly suspected at the time, 24, Belvedere Place.

But for a few, including the Fine Gael man and another eminent Irish political figure referred to always by the women as The Schoolboy, cautionary counsel seemed to act only as a spur driving them to within an inch of personal and professional disaster. Their state of mind seems remarkably similar to the personality traits found commonly in chronic gamblers in which the risk of losing is the source of the endorphine 'high' – not the risk of getting away with it, or winning, as is commonly thought. Furthermore, both men must have known better than most of the clients of the Kasbah that there would be little public sympathy, much less understanding, for men such as they who were handing over considerable amounts of their State stipend for sexual services many people in Ireland would consider immoral and vile.

A detective friend of mine who had observed the Kasbah affair closely described The Schoolboy's predicament with some sense of theatre. 'On a clear day in this country it is still possible to see Lucifer's Gates – a politician knows that better than most.'

The Schoolboy – a member of the Oireachtas, the Irish Parliament consisting of the Upper and Lower Houses – made weekly trips to the Kasbah for his caning sessions. He was a Discipline client through and through. He preferred a big girl called Georgina O'Kane because she could throw her considerable bulk into her wrists as she flailed the naked politician until he screeched in pain and orgasm. 'I very rarely had to actually touch that man,' she told me. 'He would come while he was being caned, while the blood was spilling down his legs.'

At other times The Schoolboy would ask the girls – any of the girls – to inflict the most excruciatingly painful abuse on him. One of his nipples is stretched beyond non-surgical repair as a result of this procedure.

Georgina and Linda Lavelle were the recognised specialists amongst the Discipline clients. The difference in attitude to the job between the two women who were similar in size and age was remarkable. Linda appeared to have a real concern for her clients – a concern about the way they would receive her violence – and a kind of detached liking for what she would inflict upon them in the way of pain and humility.

Georgina, on the other hand, set about her task with brutality and barely concealed anger.

Linda referred to all her customers, including the ones interested in Discipline, as clients. Always clients. Georgina never used the word and when I once asked her about this she replied, 'Clients, yeah, clients me arse. What do you think I am, a fucking doctor? They're all mad bastards. They're pathetic mad bastards.'

In the summer of 1991 The Schoolboy invited two of the Kasbah girls – Georgina and Mandy Jameson – to a picnic high in the Dublin Mountains overlooking an area in the neighbouring county of Wicklow which still holds some remnants of old British colonial rule. 'He picked us up at the Kasbah around midday and the three of us headed out,' said Georgina. '"My treat," he said. "I owe you girls a treat."'

The sun was blazing down as The Schoolboy took a hamper out of the back of his car and laid out the wine, caviar, smoked salmon, the plates, the stemmed glasses, the whole show. 'It was like something out of those old British television programmes where the Lord and Lady of the Manor head off for a day in the country in their Rolls Royce. The Schoolboy was acting like our own personalised butler!' said Mandy.

After settling the girls in nice and comfortably on a soft tartan rug spread over the lush green sward, The Schoolboy went to the back of the car again and took out a wooden kitchen chair, a long piece of rope and a towel and began to take his trousers and underpants off, leaving his vest, shirt and socks in place. Said Mandy, 'He asked me to tie him up "good and fucking tight", good and fucking tight is what he said, and then to continue on scoffing the wine and caviar while he watched. Of course we did it. Linda had trained us well and once you're with a client you should always expect the unexpected and go along with it. Our client had planned this all along as a session and we had to go into roles as soon as he let us know what he required. It's our bread and butter.' In this case, of course, it was their wine and caviar. The Schoolboy was tied fast to the chair, eyes fastened to the clear blue sky, as the girls resumed their five-star nosebag.

In a metamorphosis which owed more, perhaps, to some unknown Oedipal catastrophe than anything else more obvious, the ladies' client started to whimper from his incarcerated position like some little boy lost. 'Please, please can I have some food. I'm terribly hungry. And please, please, don't hit me. Don't hurt me.' Mandy knew the signals straight away; she knew what her client required.

'Shut the fuck up over there, you little cunt. Shut the fuck up or I'll take a stick to you.'

'Oh please don't do that!'

'I'm fucking warning you, now. Shut the fuck up while we're eating.'

'I just want a little bit of food. I'm *so* hungry.'

'Right. Right, you little bollocks, you asked for it.'

Mandy and Georgina found a small wooden switch and began the awful rite of Discipline. The hungry boy-man politician howled in pain and pleasure before ejaculating into the blood running down the inside of both legs. Minutes later he was untied in silence, quickly and professionally by two women who had lost their stage anger as instantaneously as they had found it. They made sure not to look him in the eye, knowing his profound embarrassment right at that moment. He quickly cleaned himself down with the towel as the two women busied themselves bundling what was left of the picnic into a wicker basket.

'Very good', he said, his strong masculine voice now fully restored. 'Very good. Can I give you girls a lift into town?' Three hundred pounds was given over there and then: the usual rule of asking for the readies beforehand would not have been appropriate this time because it would have punctured the fantasy. (Anyway, Georgina explained later, The Schoolboy could be relied upon to pay money – good money – without quibble.)

The Schoolboy took the cash out of his wallet and handed

it over as if he were paying a mechanic for doing a good job on his car . . . or was he, I wondered as I was being told the story, paying for something else, something beneath the surface like a sad and emotionally empty little boy he had just revisited? Maybe the nickname given to him by his whores suggested that they understood this man better than I ever would.

He drove his two women servants into town. As usual, politics or some such other non-sensitive issue was chosen for conversation. And as ever with Slaves and Discipline clients, eye-to-eye contact would not be resumed until the next session.

The Schoolboy had been a client of the Kasbah for almost the ten years of its existence. None of the women from that place could remember a single encounter with him involving straight sex. 'He loved being a naughty, bold little boy,' recalled Linda. 'The "naughty boy" thing was his sole reason for being in the Kasbah. Very often he would come to the Kasbah and announce like a schoolkid that he'd no money. The girls would then have to search his pockets: they'd only find small change and they'd chide him for this. Of course it was an act. He was getting his rocks off being searched. He always looked for reasons to be punished. He would require to be punished – disciplined – for having no money. He would never pay us less than £200 at the end of any session.'

Linda remembers his first visit to the Kasbah some nine years earlier.

'He arrived one night for a Discipline session and he was out of luck because we'd heard that there were police raids taking place on the brothels at the time and we got all the whips and chains and bits of leather gear out of the way just in case. Then Vikki had a great idea. She offered to tie him up in the flex of the vacuum cleaner which he agreed to. We gave him a right good hiding, a real bad beating and he started to moan like a whipped pup. This annoyed Vikki who wasn't, at that time, all that used to the Discipline clients. "Shut the fuck up," she said to him. "Shut the fuck up or do you see this," she said showing him the three-pin plug on the end of the cable, "D'ya see this. I'll plug this in somewhere and we'll all have a right good fucking groan!'"

Like The Schoolboy, the Fine Gael man may have been at the mercy of the prostitutes of the Kasbah during their hours together, but he was no little boy lost when it came to surviving outside those fantastic environs. After being caught on police surveillance camera entering and leaving 60B Mountjoy Square West, he was approached by detectives and asked to accompany them to Fitzgibbon Street police station to make a full statement. They told him about their video-taped evidence, which revealed the registration number of his car, the frequency of his visits, etc. Unlike thirteen similarly compromised clients who gave depositions, he refused to make a statement, although cautioned that not to do so could result in police calls to his house as part of routine enquiries into the case. He gave just his name and address – all that was required under the law. (He was probably more aware than most that the video evidence alone was more show biz in nature than police biz. The fact that 123 men were caught on camera entering and leaving premises suspected of being a brothel, could never on its own have made the case of brothel-keeping or brothel-managing: it would have been inconceivable to use such material as main evidence in court.) The thirteen of the Fine Gael client's confrèers who gave signed statements of having received sexual services for money at the Kasbah later had their 'confessions' accepted into evidence in the lower courts: their necks were now firmly on the public chopping block especially when it became known that Marion Murphy was going to contest the charges brought against her.

The Fine Gael man's involvement in the world of paid vice did, however, become a public issue when the fact that he had been caught on video surveillance was highlighted in the newspapers. There was public outcry over the leak and the police were blamed in some of the newspapers for it. Tensions were heightened to near fever pitch at one point when one newspaper was actively considering raising the ante by naming the politician involved.

As usual, there was not a squeak of outrage recorded over the fact that the clients themselves were never put in the firing line for legal reprimand and that officialdom had invested so much energy in concealing their identities.

The Fine Gael client has since become vulnerable and discredited among many of his peers as a result of the whole affair. He still regularly visits the girls for his Discipline sessions, although his sojourns have been less frequent since he became aware that research was being carried out for a book about the Kasbah. He telephoned Linda Lavelle at her home only three days after Marion Murphy was convicted of brothel keeping offering his heart-felt sympathies and concern for her future and that of Linda's family. In the same conversation he made an appointment to see her later on that week for a Discipline session.

Linda recalled her feelings when she put down the phone. 'I thought to myself, "Well fuck him. He really doesn't give a shit." He promised to come up with a big, fine legal plan when Marion Murphy was charged. He promised to help us all out after the police raid [on the Kasbah] but he just vanished into thin air and now he telephones me offering me sympathy and really looking for me to look after him, you know, as a client. Dave, are you going to name him in the book? Name the fucker. He is not really with us at all.'

The issue of whether to name the Fine Gael client in this book along with other public as well as lesser known clients, serves more than any other factor to pin-point the complex personality of Linda Lavelle. Initially, she was prepared to name 'every fucking one of them': in the days after the Circuit Criminal Court case she had decided to post to the homes of the thirteen State's witnesses their signed depositions of having received sex in the Kasbah, copies of which she had managed to get from the defendant's Book of Evidence. She only refrained from this course of action at the time because of how it might have been viewed in the event of Marion Murphy appealing against the court ruling. Linda Lavelle was – and still is – ambivalent about naming the Fine Gael client, The Schoolboy, the leading churchmen, lawyers, the high-flyer in the GAA, and, of course, the police clients who were still on her books.

The fact that she was prepared to name her errant men under the right circumstances has much more to do with a perceived sense of betrayal than any malice. Said Linda Lavelle, 'Marion Murphy found herself alone sitting in the dock, named in the newspapers, for three whole days for the whole world to see while a little arrangement between the judge and the lawyers meant that the clients' identities were never revealed. That's not justice, that's not fair. Maybe I should name them if no one else will.'

Both Linda and the other prostitutes of the Kasbah make the further disturbing claim that the depositions read out in court by the clients caught on video bore little resemblance to what most of them really got up to at the Kasbah. 'They perjured themselves. The GAA man, for instance. He was the most dirty, rotten horrible pervert bastard in the business yet his statement to the cops tells of him going into the Kasbah for a straight ride! That man wouldn't know what to do with a straight fucking ride.'

For the moment at least, she has not put the thirteen depositions in the mail box to the families of the men who were once her clients as she has often threatened to do. 'I want the people out there, I suppose I want the women out there, to know what some of these men are really doing when they visited the Kasbah. I want the women of Ireland to know what's going on, I suppose.'

I remember thinking to myself at the time that if there was

any wickedness in Linda Lavelle it was a wickedness borne of a mischievous enjoyment of doing the wrong things, illicit things, things with men that were outside the normal confines of acceptable behaviour, men whose needs and desires are both strange and repulsive to most of us, but understood and met by Linda Lavelle and her women of the Kasbah. Despite her shocking stories and despite my better efforts, I could find nothing within this woman that was personally repulsive, wrong or objectionable.

Chapter Eight

Of Werewolves And Slaves

The Fine Gael man and The Schoolboy were not the only politicians to frequent the Kasbah in its early years. Neither were they the most extreme in their proclivities to the outer edges of sexual behaviour. One of the main contenders for that ghoulish honour must surely belong to a TD and staunch member of the Fianna Fáil Party who was known to the girls one and all by the descriptive but unflattering title of the Fat-Assed Slave. Unlike his Parliamentary colleagues who became surprised police interviewees during the 1980 raid in Harold's Cross, the F.A.S. was a long-term 'specialist' patron of the Kasbah: as his pseudonym implied, he was not into straight sex but Discipline, Discipline at its most obsequious. 'The girls used to hate to see him arriving at the Kasbah,' said Linda Lavelle. 'They really hated it. He would come in mumbling under his breath about wanting to kiss our feet, then he would head straight to the linen room and look for a pair of the girls knickers to wash. We called him the Fat-Assed Slave because he had such an enormous arse. He had an arse like a big woman.'

Like all Slaves, the F.A.S. could be trusted. 'Trust is enormous and total with all Slaves,' said Linda 'He washed all the dirty linen for us. And in the winter he would come in before the Dáil [Irish Parliament] sessions opened in the mornings and shovel up spadefuls of coal and get the fire started. We told him to put the coal in a bucket but he preferred to bring it all the way in from the shed out the back through the hall and into the front room with a tiny shovel. The man was a total looper.' After getting the fire going, the F.A.S. would, if required, run errands to the shops for the girls, buying tea, biscuits, milk and so on, before making his way again across the city to the Government Buildings in Kildare Street and into the heady corridors of power where his female secretary would be at hand to brief him on the tasks that lay ahead during the day's sitting. Whenever he got the opportunity, he would make his way back to his wonderland of powerlessness across the River Liffey in Mountjoy Square West where he would collect the girls' ill-gotten gains in time to make giro deposits in their various bank accounts.

'Trust is enormous and total . . .'

The Fat-Assed Slave remained true to role even when he accidentally bumped into Linda in a hotel dining room in one of the Border counties in 1985. 'I was with my mother and father and I nearly died when I saw him come through the doors with an entourage of people. I asked myself what he was doing up here in this neck of the woods? He's not from this part of the country – he has no ties here at all. Then I thought, I hope he doesn't call me Madam or something like that in front of my mother and father!'

Nothing of that sort happened – although Linda had good grounds for her anxiety – for it was Madam Linda Lavelle, as distinct from her Kasbah Health and Fitness Studio light years away in Dublin, who was the spark that ignited the F.A.S. into his sexual subservience. From the moment he caught sight of her, he kept a discreet and innocent looking distance, playing host to a table of party faithful which he held together with handsome authority during this visit to a constituency far away from his political home base . Only when Linda and her parents got up to leave did the F.A.S. show any signs of his 'role', interrupting the proceedings at his own table as he dashed for the dining hall door to open it for Linda, shifting right past her in the process and past her again in time to open the main entrance door. Not a word from him. Just unquestioning subservience.

'Trust is enormous and total . . .'

Linda's mother asked her who that nice courteous man was as they made their way across the car park. 'Oh, he's just some TD looking for a bloody vote. They're all the same, mama.' All the time Linda was thinking, 'Oh Jesus, mama, if you only knew . . .'

The symbiosis between Slaves and the prostitutes they choose to serve appears inviolable. 'Part of their turn-on is being given the trust and fulfilling it,' said Linda Lavelle. 'Slaves could be the biggest gangsters going, could be Mafia bosses. But once the prostitute he's dealing with – the girl he takes punishment from – is good at her job and has him under control she could trust him with her life-savings and he would guard it for her with his life. Only the other day I gave a Slave £500 to deposit in a bank account. The branch had been moved to another street but he found it and came running back to me with the receipt. He was so pleased with himself. He was like a little boy who had done well in the shops for his mammy. You couldn't trust another type of client with anything like that.'

Despite his hopeless and complete servility, the F.A.S. was no less vulnerable to the knife when it came to the ridicule and cruelty the prostitutes at the Kasbah could mete out on occasions. He was about to find this out at huge cost to his dignity on one Friday night in 1985 as he tucked his Parliamentary Questions papers away in his briefcase and headed out into the cold night air from the warmth of Buswells Hotel – a favourite watering hole of Irish parliamentarians and their hangers-on – and took off on foot to his fantasy land across the city.

Mandy recalls the day as having been a busy one for the girls at the Kasbah. 'I mean really busy. We made a fortune from eleven o'clock that morning and we decided to have a piss-up in the Kasbah. There were four of us there at the time and we sent word to two other girls in a massage parlour nearby. We closed shop early [10.30pm to 11pm was the loosely observed closing time every night of the week] and got locked out of our skulls on vodka and wine.'

In their carefree abandon to the transports of ethyl alcohol, the girls forgot to switch off the lights in the front room: the almost imperceptible radiance through the heavily-set curtains was a long-established code sign to clients and would-be clients on the outside that the girls were open for business. At 10.45pm there was knock on the door which was answered by Ann Charlton (not her real name), a diminutive soft-spoken woman with a high voltage temper. Probably for the first time, they were pleased to see the F.A.S. standing there, ruddy-faced and whiskey-breathed, in all his sartorial elegance. 'Come in, won't you. Come in and have a drink with us,' said this spider to this fly. One hour later this man of considerable political substance was turning his head in search of his clothes, still smarting from the unusually enthusiastic Discipline session administered in turn by three of the drunken women. His legs were bloodstained front and back, as were the tumbling flesh folds of his large behind. 'Parts of him looked like a fucking unbaked pizza!' Ann told me later.

For the girls, however, the party had only just begun. It was with unconscionable and gutsy delight that they retold the story for me. 'Where's my clothes?', The Fat-Assed Slave asked no one in particular. Mandy was never short of answers to questions like that. 'Here, you mad fucker, here's your tie. The rest is going to cost you money.' With that, the girls descended on him, grabbing an arm, a leg, and whatever other point of leverage was available, and in Mandy's words, 'We fucked him out on the street; he was black and blue, with the blood running out of his arse. He was begging for his clothes back but we were shouting "No way, José, where's the fucking money?" We were all laughing like fucking hyenas!'

Luckily for the F.A.S. he had more than the £100 cash the girls had taken off him for the Discipline session and after a while managed to re-purchase his unwittingly mortgaged sober grey suit and accessories. Bowed and bloodied, he dressed himself on the pavement and got back to the Dáil to collect his car and make his long and very painful trip back home to his political constituency. One of the girls in his other constituency of perversion in the Kasbah that night was Pia Masterson. She later reflected, 'unlike any other brothel I have ever worked in, when a Discipline client like the Fat-Assed Slave came in we'd all get involved and have a laugh, even though the client would never know we were laughing at him. It got a bit out of hand that night when we threw him out on the street. He'll know better than to come without an appointment the next time!' And she excused the collective behaviour of the women that night thus, 'Look, if you didn't have a laugh, if you didn't get a high in this business you'd go mad. Totally off the head mad.'

And it appeared to be more than mere happenstance that both the Fat-Assed Slave and the two TDs caught literally with their trousers down in the 1980 raid in Harold's Cross Road were paid up members of the Fianna Fáil Party. 'It's peculiar, you know, when the Fianna Fáil Ard Fheis [the party's annual conference] is on in Dublin,' said Linda Lavelle, 'that's very big money for us and other prostitutes in the city. We're all out in force when the Fianna Fáil men are in town for a shindig. I once asked a teacher client of mine called Jack [not his real name] who was also in Fianna Fáil why they were so into it and paying . . . and yet the Fine Gael [the main opposition party] were not. He told me, "It's funny, you know, Linda, that after the conference is over the Fianna Fáil lads are all in at the bars slugging down their large whiskeys but the Fine Gael men are sipping tea and eating sandwiches in the anterooms. They're from different backgrounds. It's a cultural thing."'

Linda Lavelle surmised, 'Whatever the reason, the Fianna

Faíl men are mad into the ladies. Fine Gael-ers aren't worth a shite for business.'

Neither Linda or her teacher friend held any such bias when it came to members of the Labour Party. One such member was a frequent client of the Kasbah where he took a liking to Pia. He was the man the women referred to as The Full Moon TD. Pia explained, 'He was a really pleasant type of fella and for a long time he was in the newspapers nearly every night of the week. He always made a phone call to the Kasbah and collected me well away from the place. We'd drive off in his car out of town to some hotel car park or somewhere like that and I'd hold his prick: that was all. He just talked about family problems, the wife, the kids, the usual stuff and I'd sit there in the front seat and listen while I was holding his willy. Now and again he'd ask me to pull him off, you know, to wank him, but that was rare enough.'

Each time they made their way out to the Labour man's car park confessional, Pia would have one eye to the night sky. She knew if there was a full moon she was going to earn her money. 'Jesus, it was a scream. Once there'd be a full moon the man would lose his fucking reason altogether. He'd be roaring like a wolf I swear to God. He'd be looking out the window at the moon and roaring like a fucking wolf! And he'd have me on me all fours on the seat and he'd be trying to take the knickers off me with his teeth, roaring all the time. He was like a fucking werewolf. He'd be roaring and trying to get on top of me and eating me knickers. Jesus, you knew you'd been out on a job after one of those nights.'

There was no such client profile for men of the cloth. Almost without exception, they are the most loathed of all the prostitutes' clients.

Initially, I had wrongly and naïvely assumed that the prostitutes' obvious dislike of the clergy had something to do with the guilt they must feel as 'fallen women', and that this feeling was somehow amplified during their sinful rites with the religious. There is no doubt in my mind that, with some exceptions, the vice trade women are by and large not in love with their carnal profession, but most of them seem able to handle it at some level, either by will-power or straight acceptance of their own behaviour. Few if any of the prostitutes, however, find these tools of survival very effective against verbal abuse – the one trait common to nearly all their clerical clients. And it is this form of abuse rather than any heightened sense of humiliation which makes the prostitutes cringe at having to 'look after' their very considerable clientele of priests of every rank in the Irish hierarchy.

One such man is Father Pat (not his real name), also known to the women of the Kasbah as The Whispering Priest because of his disposition to speaking in tones more appropriate to the confessional. Vikki, in particular, had taken strong personal dislike to this middle-aged guardian of the moral and spiritual welfare of his flock who holds a position of some eminence in the church to this day. Once, after a session in which he made his payment in the usual manner, by way of personalised cheque issued from a Dublin city bank with his bona fide identity clear for any of the prostitutes who would care to examine it, she asked him how he would respond if a parishioner woman asked him for one or two pounds to feed her children. It was a question, I discovered, that provided its own insight into a period of Vikki's life when, as a child, her mother was frequently required to seek alms from the Church and other institutions in order to provide for her children. Vikki told me, 'He didn't bat an eyelid, Dave. As quick as a shot he told me that he would give her a bloody good lecture about wastefulness and greed and here's me talking to him and holding a cheque in me hand for a couple of hundred quid for screwing him and taking his abuse. He'd tell her to stop smoking cigarettes or whatever and cut out needless spending and to manage her money better.

'He then said he would give her the couple of quid and send her on her way.'

Chapter Nine

Money And Motive

Three powerful figures in the Roman Catholic Church availed themselves of the sexual services of the prostitutes at the Kasbah according to the accounts given to me by four of the women who worked there. Before setting out their stories in detail, I feel it is appropriate to examine why this book came into existence in the first place; why Linda Lavelle and women like her decided to allow a journalist like me to enter this most secret world with a view to writing a book about it and why their stories should be believed.

Firstly, the project was never about financial gain for either Linda or the other prostitutes. When we started discussing the nitty gritty of possible publishing deals, Linda and her partner Liam wanted to know how much money I needed to launch the book! (I remember one startling occasion in their home in late 1993 when I raised the question of money. The pair turned and looked at each other before Linda asked, 'How much do you need to get started? We'll be able to contribute [financially] to the book. I'm not talking a lot, now, Dave. I won't give you £10,000, but I'll give you enough to get started on it.')

After a time we agreed on a percentage 'cut' of the royalties. And once the decision was made not to name the clients whose depositions were largely responsible for bringing about the court case in February 1993, her attitude to the whole project changed markedly, making it clear that she wanted no monetary gain at all. In effect, she had distanced herself from the book, yet she encouraged me to continue to create it. 'I just couldn't allow myself to be seen as part and parcel of this book as an authorised biography without naming names,' she once told me, explaining, 'it's the underdogs like me and the girls and even Little John Keegan who keep being named while the others are still protected.' The many prostitutes whom I interviewed, including those who had paid sex with the three major Church figures have no monetary investment in this book whatsoever and have received no payments for the countless hours they have given during its compilation.

Linda Lavelle's decision, and, through her, the decision of the other prostitutes, to meet me and reveal the secrets of their trade – their lives – is one, I suspect, which I do not even partially understand. At early stages of the research, during the interviews and the constant telephone calls made in the process of checking and double checking, the motive looked clear enough: it was a simple act of vengeance against men, everyone from Little John Keegan to those who peopled the judiciary and the police force and, to a slightly lesser extent, the clients of the Kasbah. But that motive appeared to me to evaporate when my reluctance to write a book that named names became evident.

It was at that point – sometime in the autumn of 1993 – that I first discerned that Linda Lavelle had become more interested in me as a person than in the book I was writing. 'Look,' she told me, 'maybe the book is not a good idea as far as I'm concerned. Maybe I should have waited until I retire or leave the country. I know the effort you have put into it and I want you to go ahead with it but can you do that, Dave, without using my real name? Would that destroy the whole thing for you?'

She would further explain, 'Just look around me, Dave. Liam. The kids. My parents. Me father and mother couldn't take it . . . a book. Are you very disappointed? What do you think? Can you write it without using my real name? Will it be too weak and watery if you do that? Will anyone believe it?' (I later discovered that her father was more robust than I had been led to believe. He was dead set against Linda's involvement in the book *unless* every name that could be named was named! He had argued with her that she owed it to herself to lift the lid on her betrayers and if I was not prepared to do that then she should have little or nothing to do with the project.)

How was I to interpret this and respond to Linda's concerns? I guessed that if I had pushed the matter she would have given way and consented, no matter how reluctantly, to the use of her real name. The thing that was stopping me was that I knew she was right; that a book such as this – a story such as hers – was something she and her family would need protection against if their identities were revealed, protection I could not supply. There was also the undertaking I had made to both Linda and Liam from the outset that they had the final say in matters such as the use of their own names.

More importantly, Linda Lavelle was by now regarding me as a friend rather than as a journalist she could trust. Even during her most profound misgivings about the book, there was never any indication that she expected me to call a halt to the whole thing. 'I wouldn't want you to stop now,' were words she had spoken to me a score of times. 'That wouldn't be fair on you. It's your book and I hope you make a million out of it. You deserve it. It's just the names: can it be done without our names being published?' And she would add, 'Are you browned off with it, Dave? Is Mary [my wife] fed up with it going on for so long? Does she mind me ringing your house? I bet she thinks there's other things you could have chosen to write a book on!'

The answer to why the accounts of the prostitutes of the

Kasbah should be believed is not a straightforward one. Few sections of society can have less credible character profiles than the women who prostitute their bodies for the sake of financial gain. Conversely, many of the men they served and continue to serve have distinguished themselves by scaling the highest peaks of moral and intellectual excellence: the task, therefore, of dismissing the stories of these women and by extension this book, is an easy one on the face of it.

To go that route, however, would be to ignore facts that are already part of the public domain. It's a fact that thirteen clients were called to give evidence and gave sworn depositions in front of the District Court admitting that they had sexual services in return for money. The argument also ignores the very existence of the Kasbah and what it provided during a ten year period.

Significantly, a dismissal of these accounts holds within it the notion of selective credibility. Who would have believed Annie Murphy over the Bishop Eamonn Casey affair, for instance, were it not for the child she had had by him? Who would have believed the prostitute's word over the leading figure in the GAA had he not implicated himself to the police? Who would have believed a whore in basement brothel rather than the medical doctor, known for his altruistic work with a variety of underprivileged sections of the community, were it not for a similar event? Who, indeed, would have believed the prostitutes in the face of persistent denials from the Fine Gael politician were it not for the police video that clearly indicated his familiarity with the basement of 60B Mountjoy Square West, the Kasbah?

For me, there is a much more compelling reason for believing. It is in the women themselves and the manner in which they told me their stories. There were no rehearsals; no conspiracies. The prostitutes of the Kasbah and other massage parlours knew each others' clients intimately simply because they talked about them all the time while on their shifts, especially during the quieter moments of their working days and nights. One prostitute, Joanne Kelly (not her real name), put it eloquently, 'I must have known nearly all the important clients in the game.' She gestured with her hands floating away from her chest in a movement which looked strangely balletic. 'I can't speak for the other girls but it was a way for me of getting the clients out of my head, of giving them away a bit so that I don't have to live alone with them in my head. We always talked about them during our spare time at the brothels. It was more like a laugh than telling secrets. There are no secrets in this game. It's just a thing we did. Like, when we'd be off duty and meet up for a drink there was an unwritten rule that we never discussed our clients. It was like it was a different world.'

Linda Lavelle was listening in and was at that time more bullish about the book, and she was always more fundamentalist than Joanne. 'It's time the Irish people knew the truth about their churchmen and their lawyers and politicians and businessmen. It's time people knew exactly what went on in the Kasbah.'

Chapter Ten

Sins Of The Cloth

Mandy Jameson had planned to stay well to the back of the church during the sacrament which would confer on her twelve-year-old son the holy sacrament of confirmation. 'I was never one for churches. I'm not a regular Mass-goer or anything like that.' She wasn't overjoyed, therefore, when her brother-in-law rang at the last minute to say he couldn't act as sponsor to the lad because of a sudden sickness and she would have to step in herself. Mandy was already anxious enough that morning, suffering from a mind-snapping hangover and knowing that three of her aunts – nuns – would be in the congregation to lend their curious form of moral support which she always interpreted as more to do with intrusive and patronising nosiness. The three Sisters did that sort of thing, especially for their Mandy. She strongly suspected that, even at this impossible juncture in her life, the three holy women would be praying that a reconciliation might still be possible between herself and the husband she had almost killed all those years before.

In keeping with Roman Catholic custom and tradition, the local bishop was on hand to administer the sacrament. The boys and girls dressed in miniature men's suits and bridal-like lace and finery respectively were led to the altar by their sponsors, Mandy's slightly shaky hand on her lad's shoulder. She had her eyes on the ground until the very point at which tradition demanded that she raised them – the point where the bishop confirms his new acolyte to the Church. Mandy froze in horror and disbelief as she looked around at the many clerics, including the church figure who was about to aid her son's passage into adult spiritual existence. For among these holy men was the man she had slept with for £200 only two nights earlier. 'I remember thinking, "This just can't be fucking happening. This is not fucking real. Beam me up, Scotty, for Jesus' sake."' The churchman didn't flinch. He looked straight into her face and carried on with his role in the religious passage being enacted. The three nun aunts kneeling in the pews in their identical black habits some way back were silent in prayer. Only Mandy, her clerical client and the Being they were all there to exalt could have known of their subterranean alliance in a basement in Mountjoy Square West so far removed from this house of God.

The churchman in question was and still is a reviled character in the world of prostitution for two reasons. 'His language was atrocious,' said Mandy. 'He would always ask "What are you?" when he was riding you and answer his own question with, "a fucking whore, that's what you are." Then he would say, "what am I doing in a place like this screwing a fucking whore?"'

'Other times,' she said, 'he would talk about tearing the arse off me, about me being a dirty little whore, only a prostitute, only a fucking little cunt. Those were the words he always used and yet to see him up there during the confirmation; fuck me, someone should know what's really going on . . .'

This churchman had a taste for being, as Linda Lavelle euphemistically put it, 'very personal': he took liberties from the prostitutes of the Kasbah that were never up for sale. 'He was into touching up and French kissing. He would not want a girl unless she was very personal,' said Linda. 'And he would always look for young girls. I have seen young prostitutes come out from the room after being with this particular client and they'd be crying their eyes out from his filthy talk.'

The churchman's willingness to part with his money maybe made things a little less repulsive for his women servers at the Kasbah. In the sometimes hardened words of Linda Lavelle, 'When you're at the game for a while you just tell yourself that this man is paying for it like the rest of them and blank out what sort of abuse you're getting for it.' Unlike whispering Father Pat and his personalised cheques, this churchman went to extraordinary lengths to conceal his identity and rank within the Church from the prostitutes. Prior to each visit to the Kasbah he would purchase a shirt and jumper which he would put on sometime shortly before he arrived for his session. While he was getting dressed after sex in one of the back rooms he would tell the girls that he was carrying out research into a specialist area in one of the sciences, and one in which he appeared to have some expertise. He had been a client at the Kasbah for eight years before any of the girls knew who he really was: until that day when Mandy looked up from the sacred marble floors of the church to see him taking part in the rites of confirming her son. A short time later, Linda and her partner Liam were at a public show in Dublin when they bumped into the same cleric. 'He had a long coat on him and was chatting away to two very well-groomed women,' she recalled. 'It's only when I looked down and saw his priest's smock or whatever you call it that he realised I knew he was a clergyman. He nearly fucking died!'

Many of the prostitutes I had spoken to believed that the behaviour of their male clients in brothels represented a reversal – a complete reversal – of the roles they acted out in their public lives. Joanne Kelly is one such believer. She is a strikingly handsome woman in her mid twenties. She is both tall and elegant. She has dark cropped hair and large brown eyes, a favourite and often favoured prostitute among her contemporaries, and one whom another powerful figure in the Roman

Catholic Church in Ireland had much time for. He was never a client of the Kasbah, but he paid ex-Kasbah girl Joanne for sex and was a frequent visitor to another so-called massage parlour on the south bank of the Liffey, the river which runs through the heart of the old city of Dublin. 'He was very kinky,' she recalled. 'He became a client sometime around 1983 and was using the girls right up to late 1991.' Like the previous leading clergyman client, this one, too, was a figure of detestation and contempt among the parlour girls. Said Joanne, 'He used to say, "You're being fucked now, girl, you're being rightly fucked now, me lass," as he was going on top of me.'

This Church figure made some efforts to conceal his identity, but he certainly wasn't obsessive about it. He would arrive at the parlour at the preappointed time in trainers, corduroy slacks, a shirt and jumper. He only showed nervousness, according to Joanne, whenever conversation rushed to fill the vacuum created when he and his prostitute were dressing themselves after having sex. 'He wouldn't like being asked any questions,' she said. 'He made gruff sorts of replies which didn't mean anything. They weren't words at all.'

The churchman would require one final gesture from his prostitute before leaving his coital den. 'Every time we were finished and dressed he would ask me to kneel down and kiss his hand,' she said.

What this somewhat secretive cleric never knew was that his identity had long since lost its interest and newness for the girls. A security video system in the parlour ensured that no secrets, none of these poignant, pathetic moments of a deeply troubled and selfish man, could he regard as private and he had long since become the butt of waspish jokes among the prostitutes gathered at the television monitor in a 'staff only' room. When it comes to strychnine-laced invective and sarcasm, few sections of society could stay in the ring with the ladies of the bordellos for longer than a couple of rounds.

'Did you kiss his hand today, Joanne?'

'Did he kiss yours!'

'"You're being rightly fucked now, me lass!"'

'You're right there, you horny old bastard.'

'Kiss my fanny you fucking pervert.'

'I must go to Confession and tell the priest that [the client] wanted to kiss my hand.'

'That'll get you a few fucking Hail Marys and a lash of the Rosary.'

There were no such hidden prying eyes in the rooms used by the third powerful Church figure. Unlike his colleagues, there is no evidence to suggest that he ever entered one of the seedy massage parlours flourishing in Dublin at the time. For he was the take-away cleric, the man who, three or four times every month, lifted the telephone from his expensive hotel suite in Dublin where he was booked in with his male sidekick and sought room service – on an outside line.

If questions of moral value should ever be asked of the clerics who preach one life and, for some of the time at any rate, practise another, they should surely be asked of this man. For not only was he a seasoned campaigner in the world of hired sex in Dublin (and beyond), he was also something of an inveterate cannabis smoker during his carnal clinics in the hotel suite.

It was no accident that he took an immediate liking to Vikki O'Toole: one of her glorious weaknesses is for alcohol and her precious 'wacky baccy' or marijuana joints. (Time and time again during the compilation of this book she failed to turn up for interviews scheduled for late morning. We would make contact later in the day: 'Jesus, Dave I'm sorry. I do be strung out in the mornings, luv. Any chance can you do the interviews of an afternoon? I do have me head on me in the afternoons.' Vikki burns it, some would say literally, at both ends. But despite everything, it's impossible not to love this most shocking and amoral of women.)

The churchman would always phone Linda Lavelle in the

Kasbah shortly after checking into one of Dublin's more fashionable and expensive hotels. More often than not he was accompanied by another man who was not a priest of the Church. Over the phone he would use his code name and ask Linda for two girls to be sent to his hotel, room number such and such. He would almost always ask for Vikki and insisted that she bring the cannabis. Said Vikki, 'I would go along there with another girl and we would sit in the room all night just having sex and smoking 'blow'. He might start off riding me and then turn to whatever girl I brought along. The two of them took turns in screwing us which was okay. But he was a crude bastard. When he'd be on top of me he'd be saying things like, "Get that into you, you fucking slut" and, "Can you feel that, bitch. Can you feel that inside you?" I didn't give a fuck to be honest because I'd be out of the game on the blow and he was a good man to pay money. I also made a bit of profit on the gear [cannabis] so I was fairly happy about the whole arrangement.'

The relationship between this churchman and Vikki soured when she arrived one night in the hotel room and explained to her patron that she was unable to get the gear. 'He was fucking furious,' she recalls. 'He told me that if I ever came without it again he'd have my kneecaps blown off. I was terrified of the man after that.' (Whether or not it was within the man's province to effect such an appalling event, Vikki was the wrong type of woman to make such threats against. She had friends – friends who made a living out of consigning people to wheelchairs. What was worse, she was something of a loose cannon and would call on such people to sort things out for her without hesitation or logic.)

According to Linda Lavelle, these three wise men of the Church will never change their sexual waywardness. 'Two of them are still doing business with my girls. One of them is off the scene. One way or the other, they will come back because they always come back the same way as perverts always come back. Once a pervert always a pervert and these three men were perverts with the language they use. Bad language was their perversion, their fantasy. That will not change and they will not change.'

She fixes her thoughts for a moment on one clergyman who was found out in a different arena and who is currently paying his own wretched price for crimes against morality. 'What do you think of Bishop Eamonn Casey? I think that poor old cunt is finished.' She was referring to newspaper reports showing the disgraced cleric in flight from the cameras in some Mexican backwater after being tracked down by journalist and author Gordon Thomas who claimed to have conducted a pre-arranged interview with the former Bishop of Galway. Linda holds the newspaper up. 'Look at him, Dave. I mean, you're a journalist, you should be asking the questions – what did he do that was any worse than the clients I look after and all the rest of the Irish churchmen who told the world that Bishop Eamonn sinned against God. *They've* fucking sinned against God, too, haven't they? They've paid prostitutes to look after them and no one knows a thing about it. To be honest with you it's pathetic to see a poor old man [Casey] of sixty-seven years of age running down a street in a foreign land with a pair of runners on his feet. What did he do to deserve this . . . he had a screw off of a woman nearly twenty years ago and it's totally destroyed him. I don't think that that man will live much longer, he's too old for this kind of thing. I feel sympathy for him: he's after having both sides of the cow and now he's running like a chased rat down some street in Mexico in a pair of runners.'

The sympathy Linda Lavelle articulates in this instance is genuine and in it lies affirmation for me that I was right to write this book about this woman and others like her with their rough-cut and sometimes brutal honesty, which is only ever found outside the restraints of correct behaviour.

Chapter Eleven

Perverts And A Man Called Gladys

If the three wise but errant Church figures ever decided to take the road back to moral and spiritual redemption they might take some consolation from the fact that they may not have as far to travel from aberration as the likes of The Rocker, The Monkey, Transvestite Mary and a high-flying businessman known cruelly as Goo Goo Ga Gaa. And God only knows how the police would describe the scene in their official reports if these highly prized and perverted clients were ever on the premises when a raid took place.

Perverts, Linda Lavelle and her girls argued over and over again, are perverts before they ever come down the steps of the Kasbah, perversion is what brings them down. And in that statement lies both their vindication and defence. 'We don't make perverts. They come to us because we supply the service they need and if we didn't they'd get it somewhere else, possibly in Amsterdam,' said Linda Lavelle. (Some of the prostitutes do admit, however, that a number of clients began their separate careers in the Kasbah feeling fulfilled by straight sex but ending up in the stratosphere of twisted sexual endeavour.)

Goo Goo Ga Gaa is a well-known businessman based outside Dublin. He is both respected and feared in the jungle of national commerce where he stands out like a lion. His business luncheon speeches concentrate more on macho terms such as 'sweat', 'work ethic', 'the will to win' and the rugby metaphor about 'getting across the line with the ball'. He is the sort of man who, I imagined, when asked by a waitress how he'd like his steak, might just reply, 'Whip off its horns, wipe its arse and wheel it on out.' Yet it was this commercial power packer who made weekly trips to the Kasbah in order to sit on a white linen-covered table with a dummy in his mouth, a bonnet on his head and an over-sized nappy and plastic pants on his bum, all of which he brought with him neatly folded in his leather-bound briefcase, in order to chant the barely comprehensible mantra 'Goo goo, ga gaa' at prostitute women for over an hour. Said Pia Masterson, 'We'd give him five minutes to prepare himself in one of the rooms and then we'd enter. He'd be all dressed up in his baby gear. I would say, "Goo goo, ga gaa" and he would reply, "Goo goo, ga gaa". Pathetic, isn't it? He would never use any other words. He would never do anything else. Only goo goo, ga gaa.'

The infantile ritual lasted for one hour and would always involve at least two girls. On one occasion Pia was joined by a young woman who used the name Susan. She was relatively new to the business – the Kasbah business – and it was her turn to play 'mamma'.

'Talk to mamma, talk to mamma. Goo goo, ga gaa. Talk to mamma. Are we not talking to mamma today pettins, has the cat got our tongue? I can't hear you.'

'Goo goo, ga gaa.'

'There's a good little baby. Talk to mamma again, now. Say goo goo, ga gaa.'

To her credit, Susan didn't show it, but she was going mental with this oddest of routines. When Pia took over, Susan said to Linda, 'Would you get that f-u-c-k-i-n-g man out of here, he's driving me nuts. Please, Linda, would you ever fuck him out.'

Later that same evening Susan was in a doctor's waiting

room on the far side of the city with her young son when the boy crossed the room to a baby strapped in a buggy and started chortling 'goo goo, ga gaa, goo goo, ga gaa, goo goo, ga gaa' while playfully prodding the infant's nose. The lad will grow up never knowing why such an innocent expression of kindred affection warranted an unmerciful clatter on the back of his head with a plastic bag containing potatoes, frozen pork chops and a food blender.

If the businessman settled for 'goo gooing and gaa gaaing' all through his session of infantile revisitation, a man known as The Rocker was strangely mute. The Kasbah and its very capable Madam Linda had two sources through which the implements for so-called specialist clients were attained. Mostly, the men would bring back their own whips, canes, garters and gussets, dildos and chains, and readily leave them in the bordello's collection for use on other clients as well as themselves. (This also insured against such items being found under the front seat of the car, at the bottom of a wardrobe or in the filing cabinet in work by someone who might not either sympathise or understand, such as a secretary or a wife.) Linda also used the expertise of a man in a run-down part of old Dublin to fashion certain items of leather for use by either the girls or their clients.

But when The Rocker arrived at the Kasbah Linda had to resort to her own ingenuity to provide for his unique tastes. For this tall, strange-looking man with electrified corkscrew hair had only one conversation during his years attending the basement at 60B Mountjoy Square West on a three-times-a-fortnight basis. He told Linda he wanted a 'Big strong girl and a yellow rocking chair'. For half an hour he would sit in the chair at the back of the brothel while one of the girls, often Linda herself and sometimes Pia, would rock him silently. 'No words were ever exchanged,' said Pia. 'Nothing. He'd just sit there eerily and silent with his arms folded while we rocked him. He paid great money for what he was getting – £150 to

£200 for a half hour's session – but by Jesus were your arms tired after rocking him for that length of time. If you stopped at all for a breather he'd just look up at you and off you'd go again.'

The Rocker never displayed interest in anything more tactile or commonly sexual than being rocked. Like virtually all the Kasbah's perverts – and a pervert he most definitely was in the eyes of the girls looking after him – there was a feeling that he could be charged whatever he could afford to pay and he would never question it. The girls would often make the very earnest observation that there was money in them there perverts.

A far more conspicuous candidate for the description of pervert belonged to a client called Mary who called at the Kasbah once a week for eight years and who was a client of Linda's in the days when she shared a flat with Lyn Grey in the posh south city suburb of Donnybrook for a short time in the 1970s.

Mary would drive his car up from the country and park it right outside the door of the Kasbah and take out a black plastic bag from the boot. He would look for either Linda or Pia, the latter being a particular favourite. Mary was a farmer. A small, bald man in his mid fifties, he would make polite conversation as Pia showed him to one of the vacant cubicles off the hallway. Five minutes later he would present himself, complete in black shoulder-length wig, high heels and a pretty – pretty grubby, that is – black velvet evening dress. 'From that point on he'd start talking about what he thought were women's things,' explained Pia. 'He'd want to know when my period was due and how many children I had and [discuss] the dreadful price of ladies' clothes, particularly the underwear, in the shops. After a while we'd both head out to the shops together as part of the fantasy. We'd buy some cigarettes and tea and the likes. I always made sure that I'd walk at least two paces behind him. He was a fucking show and heads were always turning but it didn't seem to bother him in the slightest. Coming towards the end of the hour we'd head back to the Kasbah. I'd usually wank him off and he'd get dressed again and put his stinking old clothes in the black plastic bag and head off down to his farm in the country a happy man.'

It didn't always go that smoothly for Mary, however. Linda remembers a time when she 'looked after' him in her flat in Donnybrook and then asked him for a lift back into the city centre. Farmer Mary was a decent sort and even though the trip took him out of his way he was willing to oblige. As the pair hit Leeson Street, outside the old Pelican House Blood Transfusion Service, Mary's car phut-phutted to a halt. It was rush-hour and the patience of motorists on that Friday evening was no better than during any other weekend rush.

'The horns started blaring all over the fucking place,' said Linda. 'Mary was mortified because he was in his dress and wig with loads of red lipstick on. I told him, "No fucking way am I getting out of this car, no way am I pushing this heap. Push it your fucking self."'

Mary had little option but to stagger to the rear of the car dolled-up in his black stilettos, dirty velvet evening dress, seamed flesh-coloured tights, and to begin pushing the heaving old Peugeot estate for all he was worth. Not another frustrated motorist's horn was sounded in anger from the minute he alighted from the car, leaving the stone-faced blonde Madam still anchored in the front seat, her head bowed in mortification. Neither, for that matter, did any man, woman or undecided get out to lend assistance to this hallucinatory tea-time wonder. Transvestite Mary remained a client of Linda and her girls until the end of 1992. He is married with children. 'That's why he always kept the clothes in a bag in the boot of his car,' said Linda. 'The old car was his domain. No one else ever went near it and he knew his belongings would be safe in there.' It might also have explained why the same garments, including the underwear, were never washed in twenty years, according to his prostitute women.

Whatever traffic problems Farmer Mary caused in his time, he was at least a harmless and fairly predictable client. The same could not be said of a man they called The Sister. While much fantasy is intrinsically schizophrenic, he actually managed to sub-divide his fantasy again once he got going.

Susan Skelly (not her real name) was one of his favourites. With her he would play out the most kinky sibling scenes before turning his attentions to matters more sexually bovine with less than a few seconds' notice for the girl. 'We'd know what to do the minute he popped his baldy little head around the curtain every week,' she explained. 'I'd show him to a room and wait for five minutes before knocking on the door.' Susan was the imaginary sister he always called Fiona.

'Hello, who's there? Is that you, Fiona?'

'Yes, it's me, John. Can I come in?' [Susan enters and sits beside him on the bed. After a short while she places her hand on his leg and starts rubbing him firmly as she feigns sexual excitement.]

'Stop it, Fiona! Mumma and daddy are still in the house. Stop it right away. I'm ordering you.'

'But they've gone out, John. There's just you and me.'

'Where are they gone?'

'They're walking the dog. They won't be back for ages. Do you like my breasts, John? [Susan loosens the three top buttons on her blouse and takes his hand.] See! I'm not wearing a bra today, John.'

'Oh Fiona you shouldn't. You shouldn't. What if mummy and daddy come back? What on earth would they say?'

'They'll be gone for a long time, John. Oh John . . .' [She rips at his fly and starts fondling him.]

By this stage The Sister is about to shoot his load. He steadies himself before taking off all his clothes and enters another realm of his fantasy. 'I'm the bull!', he snorts, stomping his clenched hands on the floor and rubbing the front of his neck off the side of the bed. Susan knows the message. By this time she's naked, too, and on all-fours cowering in the corner of the tiny red-lit room in affected fear and loathing, her bum pointing upwards and due north in his direction. The bull John stares directly at himself in the huge mirror. 'I'm the bull!' he roars again before looking at Susan – the character Fiona long since consigned to the archives of his mind – 'and I'm going to bull the cow!'

Said Susan, 'You get well and truly rammed by The Sister. He even massages the bottom of my back with his hand the way a farmer or a vet rubs a cow when he's trying to get something inside it. You earn your money with that client.'

The Sister was a frequent guest at the Kasbah. Despite his two-fold fantasies, his requirements were well within the ranges of capability and acceptability among the girls at the basement bordello in 60B Mountjoy Square West. In fact, everything went at the Kasbah with approval and sometimes encouragement, with the exception of physical violence and the verbal abuse so favoured by the clerics.

And so it was with ease that the girls first opened the black door to a man who, for blindingly obvious reasons, would soon become known as The Monkey. He was a Northern Ireland businessman who made fortnightly trips to Dublin which included a half-to-three-quarter-hour stay at the Kasbah.

'He'd come in full of arrogance and business and look for me or Lis O'Brien and head straight to one of the rooms without as much as a how's your father,' explained Linda Lavelle. 'A couple of the girls would undress in the room together and while they were laying on the bed in one of the back rooms, he would take what I always thought an epileptic fit would look like. The fucking man just went berserk. He started foaming at the mouth and grunting just like a fucking ape.'

The Monkey would spend the next half an hour or so jumping around the place in primal celebration: off the bed landing on his feet and hands with the agility of an oversexed tom cat, scratching the back of his head and his scrotum, sometimes simultaneously, and going 'Uugh, ugh, eeeeaaauw!' as he eyed up either Lis or Pia or whatever woman was on shift that day. Still frothing at the mouth, he would half swing, half amble, his way over to one of the girls and start nit-picking the hair on the nape of their necks for lice. When he'd locate one of these imaginary bugs he'd hold it up to the light between his thumb and index finger before cracking it open with his teeth. Sometimes, though, The Monkey got a bit carried away, if that's the correct expression. Explained Linda, 'Part of his fantasy was to cock his leg up against the shower curtain and pretend he was pissing. Once he actually did piss but he won't do it again when I'm around.'

The Monkey paid up to £100 for his forty minutes or so of primal walkabout. Like so many of the 'specialist' clients there was no question of him having full sex with one of the prostitutes, although occasionally he would masturbate to ejaculation near the end of the session while still drooped over the corner end of a bed, his head upside down and just inches from the floor, just like his beloved monkey which could only be set free during these hours.

If there was one utterly despicable client among the Kasbah's legions it was to be found in the persona of a man inaccurately described as Creepy John The Businessman (not his real Christian name). Creepy he certainly was, but a businessman was what he wanted to be but never quite became. Publicly as well as in the private environs of hired vice, Creepy John had become a very well-known figure in Ireland during the mid-1980s and he saw himself as something of an entrepreneur even though he was bordering on financial indigence. His favourite ploy to procure women was to stand outside the city's dole exchanges, resplendent and convincing in his pinstripe suit and black leather shoes ('You can always tell a man by his shoes,' he often told the girls of the Kasbah) and watch for young women, preferably blonde young women, whom he would approach with the offer of employment.

Said Linda, 'It wasn't unusual at all for Creepy John to arrive around at the Kasbah with a young woman and tell me he's got another girl who was looking for a start. The poor things didn't have a clue. They thought he was a genuine businessman looking for staff and he was very convincing. I remember saying to one girl, "Do you know where you are? Do you know what sort of place this is? Do you know you're in a brothel, love? I think you'd better be going." The poor wee thing thought that Creepy John was working for me! I remember another poor little girl bolting for the door when she realised what sort of place she was in and John was so aroused that he set after her down the fucking street. He wanted to ride her and that was that. I told her that he had no right to bring her here and that, of course, she was free to go. I kept telling her to go. Sure the poor thing was only a girl and she was so shocked she didn't even hear me. She was so panicked.'

Other prostitutes at the Kasbah had no stomach for Creepy John, either. Said blonde-haired Charlene Robertson, 'He'd always take off his wedding ring and rub it all over me. Over my stomach and sometimes he'd even push it up inside of me. I don't mind what a client does – it's part of the territory – but when a man starts to bring in stuff concerning his marriage then it's hard for anyone to take. Other times he would insist that I wear his wife's bra or her knickers. Now there's a pervert for you.'

One of the few design errors made by Linda when she first opened the Kasbah was in the tiny rooms where most of the action took place. 'I started off with surgical couches instead of beds because they could put up with more abuse but the clients said they didn't like the look of them; they were too severe or something. Then I got in single beds which seemed to please everyone.' No one was more pleased than the manager of the bedding section of a city centre retail store where Linda had an account. She used to order a new single bed every week, such was the enthusiasm and vigour of her clients, not least the swinging Monkey. Every Monday morning the girls on the early shift would have the task of testing out the beds, among sundry other maintenance checks. Much more often than not they would cart broken headboards, springs, etc., up the stairs to a spare room and telephone the nice man in the furniture shop to make another delivery. And every few months a skip would arrive to take the broken edifices of lust off to the tip head.

Prostitutes from all over the city began bringing their children to the Kasbah when a man called Gladys arrived on the scene with his friend Bernie (not his real name) in the late 1980s.

For Gladys – that was the name he had bestowed on himself with his mother's blessing when he was seventeen years of age – was official cook, chambermaid, child minder, woman minder, man minder, part-time hooker, part-time man, part-time woman, and confidante to scores of people who either worked or just enjoyed themselves in the basement of 60B Mountjoy Square West.

He had been working in a top hotel in London with his friend Bernie when both men decided to come back to Ireland. Gladys won't go into the precise details of their departure from England, other than to declare theatrically, 'I threw it all up and I've been throwing it all up ever since.'

Initially, this odd couple moved into a flat in Belvedere Place and soon befriended the girls working at the brothel in number 24. It wasn't long before Gladys introduced himself to the women at the Kasbah just around the corner and struck up a friendship with most of them – particularly Pia Masterson and Linda Lavelle.

'Linda seemed to want me around the place. I think she was just being charitable because she knew Bernie and myself were on our uppers and needed a few bob. She used to send me out to the chipper and I'd be given £1 on every order I'd bring back for the girls on the shift.

I then started cooking for the girls. After all, wasn't I a cook, darling? I'd charge £3 for a full lunch, meat and two veg, and a fiver if the girls wanted a steak. Myself and Bernie would cook the meals in our flat in Belvedere Place and bring them around on trays. Sometimes we didn't have trays and we'd just charge around the corners with the hot dinners in front of us. I'd feel sorry for the girls – and for the lovely food I was after cooking – because they never had the fucking time to eat a meal properly. They'd sit the food on their laps and then a knock would come to the door and they'd leave the food to go cold while they looked after a client. Still, it was better for them than the chipper. It stopped them breaking out in spots!'

After a month or so, Gladys and Bernie took a flat in one of the buildings which housed the Kasbah and their symbiosis with the women downstairs was complete. The two unlikely flatmates took turns in babysitting the children of the Kasbah women in their flat upstairs while the women worked below. More often than not, they would take the kids out to shopping malls and cinemas in the city centre. 'We became part of the scheme,' said Gladys. 'Girls with girls. I had become a working girl at the Kasbah, you might say. But I never lit the fire. Don't let any of them [the Kasbah women] tell you that I ever lit the fire in the mornings because I didn't. I won't get me hands dirty for love nor money.'

He can recall only one incident of sexual apartheid during his stay at 60B. 'It wasn't from the girls or the clients, either. It was from another fellow who had a flat next to mine and was always slagging me and Bernie about being queers and what he would do to us one of these days. He was a bad piece of work. One night I was watching the television in the flat when I heard a terrible commotion in the hall outside. This neighbour of mine was having the shit kicked out of him. He was being burgled and mugged at the same time. I just walked over to the telly and hiked up the volume and pretended not to hear a word. He was getting a terrible whacking.

'He crawled over to my door after it was over and I opened it. He said, "Why didn't you help me?" and I just said, "Now, darling, you've got your answer from the queers. Now, go off and wash yourself, you're a mess", and I slammed the door shut in is face.'

Gladys' first engagement as a 'working girl' at the Kasbah (he had dabbled in prostitution elsewhere previously) was with a client he fondly if crudely calls Mick the Prick. And once again I found myself challenged by the whole notion of sexual orientation when I felt the need to ask Gladys whether client Mick was gay or straight. In the world of the Kasbah, the sexual lines and roles were never defined in my rigid terms of gay or straight; black or white; right or wrong.

'He just arrived in one day without any patience at all,' remembers Gladys. 'He just wanted to shoot his load and get out and that was that. Linda told him that all the girls were busy at the time and he got fairly annoyed so she sent him down to one of the back rooms and told him to get undressed and she'd have a girl down to him right away. She asked me to go down to Mick the Prick for a gas and I agreed. Linda can be a terrible woman! I went into the room and here was this man lying naked face down on the bed; he couldn't see my face. I said, "I'm Gladys" in me best girlie voice and he turned around and looked up at me. He knew then I was a man, and, cool as you like, he said, "Gladys, will you rub me balls?"'

'I remember feeling, "Oh, oh, oh Jesus I'm w-e-e-a-k!"'

Gladys will not stop laughing, either at himself or at others. 'Mick went in there looking for a woman and he got me. He didn't really care once he got in there. He enjoyed it, that's the main thing. And I got my money and everyone was happy. I can remember him coming back twice to the Kasbah. Up to the point where he had me – or I had him – he wanted women, but the twice that he came back he looked for good old Gladys.'

Another client, P.J. (not his real initials) from County Cork, also nailed his colours to the good ship Gladys after many years of being looked after by the Kasbah women.

'He was a dirty old man. I remember once when Linda had just put down new carpets and P.J. came in and took off his shoes and socks. You could see the trail of dirt around the new carpet. I don't think he ever washed himself. I used to tell him there was spuds growing out between his toes but he couldn't give a shite. He was just kinky – he wanted his end away and didn't care how he got it.'

On another occasion Gladys and Bernie raided the in-brothel wardrobe of a woman called Spanish Rose, a genuine Hispanic long since gone from Ireland and who delighted both herself and her clients in the sunshine satins and laces she would insist on wearing at the commencement of her once a week shift at the Kasbah. 'We got all done up. Make-up, the lot. We were sitting on the sofa with one of the other girls – I can't remember who – when a client came in and chose me to look after him!' said Gladys.

The customer, a well-off businessman, had been double-duped. For, not only had he not cottoned on to the fact that Gladys was, physically at least, a man, neither was he aware that the two were neighbours from his home town of Dundalk situated halfway between Dublin and Belfast. While Gladys was many things to many people, a diplomat was never one of them . . .

'Hey,' he said to the naked businessman lying back-up naked on a bed in one of the back rooms. 'I know you. You're[—].

'You're [—] from [—] Street. D'ya not remember me? Course you do. Heard your mother was poorly. How is she? How's the missus and kids? Keeping well? Now, [—], what's your pleasure, darling?'

'No, no,' the man on the bed gasped again, as though he had seen a ghost.

'Yes, yes, darling,' replied the neighbour in Spanish Rose's best regalia. 'Funny, the people you bump into, isn't it?'

The businessman regained enough composure to ask Gladys what he was doing in a place like the Kasbah, to which he received the reply, 'Waiting on the likes of you to come in, darling.'

These were good days for Gladys. He had, indeed, become part of the Kasbah 'scheme', going out with his friend Bernie and the prostitutes to pubs and clubs around the city and feeling a sense of security he was not used to. They were frequently being barred from the 'straight' pubs and clubs, mainly because of their outrageously camp behaviour, but they departed as they arrived: as one. 'The girls were always very good to us. If there was any hint of danger or anything like that in the pubs they would shield us and protect us. We knew that we would not come to any harm when we were with them. And if we ever needed anything – food, cigarettes, drink, even – they would always give us a loan. Me and Bernie knew that the day the Kasbah was gone we were gone, too. Back on the poverty line with not as many real friends as before.'

But it was always more than food and cigarettes and drink money. 'Now and again I had problems,' said Gladys. 'Personal problems. The girls would always sit and listen for hours to me. And they understood what was going on in my head. The Joe Soaps out on the street wouldn't have a clue and they wouldn't want to know because they have their own problems and they don't want to be bothered. The girls had their problems, too, but they would always sit and listen to me for as long as it would take, regardless of what troubles they had in their own lives. They always had time. They were always there for us. I think that me and Bernie being gay helped us relate to the girls and we all had the common bond of needing to make money.'

The feeling was reciprocal. After every client, the girls would shower in the Kasbah and dry themselves off with a towel in front of the blazing coal fire. If Gladys was there he would dry their backs and cheer them up with his quite outrageous descriptions of his social life. Whether it was his sexual orientation or his clean-cut good looks, helped on a bit by his penchant for dying his hair jet black, Gladys was a big hit with some of the girls in the Kasbah who vied with each other for his or Bernie's affections.

Linda Lavelle remembers, 'A lot of the girls were really interested in having affairs with Gladys and Bernie. Sandra [not her real name] was mad after Bernie. She started doing a line with him which didn't please her boyfriend. Then he started doing a line himself with Bernie which infuriated Sandra who told him, "I'm not screwing around in the Kasbah so that you can have all that money to bring your boyfriend out for drinks, you bastard."'

The woman who most fancied Gladys was as formidable as they come. She was called Bentha (not her real name) – the peroxide blonde with the near-perfect Scandinavian accent which had fooled many a client during her short stay at the Kasbah. Bentha was, in fact, from Ballymun, a disadvantaged high-rise suburb a few miles north of the city centre.

Gladys recalls, 'Sure the woman was a lunatic for sex. She used to lie naked in one of the rooms and call me in shouting, "Gladys! Gladys! Give me Swedish, Gladys. I laak laarge men laak you, Gladys." I just had to fucking laugh and pleaded with her, saying things like, "I can't, Bentha. I'm a woman. I'm not a fucking lesbian, Bentha, I can't do it with a woman."

'Oh, Jesus, I'm sick in the stomach from laughing when I do think of that one.'

And when it came to spleen-soaked bitchiness, Gladys had few peers. 'Bentha was a poor old dipso. She always had half a bottle of vodka in her bag. It was one of the few bulges she did have 'cos she had no tits and no teeth and fuck all a bit of style apart from the mad accent.'

Gladys's openness, his flaunting of his sexuality, was in refreshing and marked contrast to many of the clients who made their way down the steps of the Kasbah over its ten years and three months. 'I never tried to hide what I am. I wouldn't live under a threat or under any possibility of blackmail. Maybe it's got something to do with the personality God gives you. How you look on life. I was always "go forward and fuck the begrudgers" and I think that helps a lot. When I was sure of what I was – or what I wasn't! – I "outed" and gave myself the name Gladys after Gladys Knight and the Pips who were big at the time. I was 16 or 17. I decided to tell me mummy about it when the time was right. It was a scream! I remember going into the kitchen and saying, "Mammy, I've something to tell you about myself. I think you'd better sit down." She looked at me and said, "It's alright, son. I know already and I've known for years. I probably knew before you knew."'

His mother's understanding was accompanied by all the maternal support her son could have wished for in the large town of Dundalk in County Louth. 'She always stood by me,' he said. 'Always. And when there was a bit of jeering she would let the message out that if people didn't like me they didn't have to come near the place and that was the end of it. You could say she didn't give a shite about me being gay. Or you could say she didn't give a shite what people thought. I'm not sure. One way or the other, she always stood by me. Always.'

What she would have thought of his sojourn at the Kasbah may or may not have been a different matter. The basement brothel certainly had impressed Gladys.

'To think of all those people – hundreds, thousands of them – walking past on the footpath outside every day going about their lives and not having a clue of the mad life in the basement! There was never a dull moment. The Kasbah was too much. Definitely too much. I wouldn't have swapped it for anything.'

Linda Lavelle could afford the expense of the broken beds and the occasional financial sponsorship of Gladys. She could sleep easy in her bed at night. Not only was vice being good to her, it was a laugh a minute as well.

Chapter Twelve

'I'll Give You
Satan's Baby'

When a woman called Minge meets up with a Satanic pervert called the The Detective all hell is likely to break loose. On a perishing winter's night in 1986 that's precisely what happened. He had called at the Kasbah about a year or eighteen months earlier and confided to Linda that he was 'a bit different' in his tastes with, and for, women. Linda Lavelle thrived on such admissions of 'difference' and the clients who make such requests – her much beloved 'loopers'. Of course she could arrange things for The Detective – an accurate monicker for a man who has given several decades of service to the Irish Police Force as both a mid-ranking officer and later as a senior one. 'Good,' he said. 'I'll be back in about a week with my stuff.' He proved to be a punctual man – and one so disturbed that he frightened the life out of some of the most seasoned prostitutes at the Kasbah. Pia Masterson was one of them.

'The routine was to leave a client in the room for a few minutes – maybe ten – to prepare himself for the girl. With straight clients this usually meant them getting undressed,' said Pia. 'With specialist clients it could mean anything, anything could be going on inside that room. As I was about to knock on the door I smelled something strange and I asked Linda could she smell it, too. I thought no more about it and entered the room and, Mother of Divine Jesus, I nearly passed out.'

The Detective was standing in a corner of the room. He had unscrewed the light bulbs and replaced them with small altar candles. He was dressed in a plain black gown which touched the floor, with a pair of silver goblets between the fingers of his left hand which he offered out in silence to the stunned Pia. A large crucifix hung from his neck and the smell of burning incense was almost overpowering. 'Here my child,' he said in his best Draculese, 'here, have some altar wine' [it was, in fact, water]. Pia went along with the fantasy, trussed by the knowledge that scary fuckers pay big bucks, too. During their half-hour together he asked her to defecate on him; he asked her to shave his body smooth and finally, finally, he whispered in Pia's ear, 'Fuck the Virgin Mary, I want you to have Satan's baby. I'm going to give you Satan's baby.'

Brothels are not generally known for their strict adherence to traditional trade union codes such as demarcation lines and changes of work practice. 'If someone is paying and you're not in any obvious danger then in you go and do the business,' says Linda. Compensation came later in the form of a few analgesic vodka and oranges. But when Pia told Linda that never, never ever, would she have anything to do with 'that Black Magic bastard' called The Detective, the Madam knew it was time to exercise her prerogative of delegation. A relieved Pia was given rights of refusal and The Detective was about to meet his equal in depravation and outrage in a girl most of the prostitutes of the Kasbah only ever knew as the Minge.

Minge was a small, red-headed woman born on the northside of Dublin and still regarded as young by her contemporaries, having reached her twenty-eighth year. She was not particularly attractive but had 'the right looks for this game', according to Linda Lavelle who explained that the more rakish a girl looked, the more takish she appeared to the clients, and, God, did Minge look rakish. She started work in the Kasbah a year before The Detective came on the scene and from a very early stage had given a strong signal of her outrageousness when a middle-aged doctor client of the Kasbah once complained to the Madam, 'Don't give me that girl again, please, Linda.'

'Why, was she not suitable?'

'Oh she was suitable alright but not at my age,' came the exhausted reply.

Minge belonged to a minority of prostitutes who actually enjoyed sex; at least in the early years. The doctor client knew he was in for a bumpy ride when he asked her in a conversational way whether she would mind if he put it, his penis, in her ear. She replied, 'You can put it in both ears at the same time if you like, darling.' She was given the name Minge as a kind of accolade: it was a reference to her long, red pubic hair, 'just like a goat's fucking beard', she often exclaimed with pride.

The day after the first session between Minge and The Detective, Linda entered the room they had used for a routine check. She left again in a rage looking for Minge. She finally caught up with her a few days later in one of the pubs in the area. 'Did you see the state of the place – did you let that fucker shite in the room again?' Minge promised her that nothing of the sort happened, although she admitted that her client had expressed the *desire* to shite. She had shaved him in the room, alright, she further confessed, but they had then left for an 'all nighter' in a hotel in one of the city's northside suburbs.

Linda needed convincing. She was painfully aware of The Detective's taste for Scatology. It was that side of him which, understandably, led Pia to put her foot down for the first and only time in her life with a client. Linda said later, 'Very few of the girls could handle something like that. You have to be totally in control of yourself and totally professional to handle a client like The Detective. It's with clients like him that the massage parlours, particularly the Kasbah, played their real role. The girls out on the street are often backward and wouldn't have the first clue how to manage specialist clients.'

As things turned out, Minge was telling the truth, and as that truth unfolded, it did so as a reminder that fiction may often be stranger than truth – but not always. And in this case few works of fiction could be as horrid, as outrageous, and as downright hilarious.

After locking up and switching off the lights at around midnight, both Minge and The Detective, a middle-aged block of a man who was married and had a large family, headed out to a northside hotel in The Detective's car where they checked in as man and wife and retired to the guests' bar to drink for about two hours. Towards the end of their drinkathon, Minge announced that she was hungry; that it was time to go to their room and get dressed up to go out for a meal. The Detective agreed. A few minutes later they both arrived downstairs and enquired of the night porter if he knew of any suitable eating establishments in the area. The poor man wasn't able to answer them for nearly a minute. What stood in front of him will, it's a fair guess, go with him to that Great Foyer In the Sky. Minge had on two items of clothing: a man's shirt, and a tie which travelled between her slender-bordering-on-skinny legs and around the front in an unsteady knot. She wasn't even wearing shoes. The Detective looked similarly attired for eating out in just a waist-length check sports jacket buttoned at the front. Again no shoes, no nothing.

Eventually the porter mumbled incredulously, 'You're not going out now are you? It's freezing cats and dogs out there. You can't go out like that, not looking like that. Not from here.' Minge replied, 'But of course, darling, we are just on our way.' With a perfunctory nod of the head from Minge, this oddest of odd couples made their way down the steps of the hotel giggling and slipping on the iced pavement below, inured to the freezing cold by the alcohol still coursing through their veins. Their first stop was at a late shop in the village of Fairview where Minge bought some cigarettes from an elderly couple who in all likelihood would not have wanted to be informed that they were serving a high-ranking respected member of the Irish police force sporting an expansive and freshly shaved bum and his near naked prostitute as they contemplated calling the police more out of panic than complaint.

The odd couple then made their way to a kebab restaurant in another suburban village which was busy catering to locals who had made their way out of pubs at closing time. Minge walked in first and made her way to the counter. Behind her, the sound of knives and forks and boozebabble dried up in an instant to become as deafeningly silent as a country church. Minge looked behind her at the diners collectively gaping in disbelief. She turned back to the waitress and ordered two kebabs and said chirpily, 'Chilly tonight, isn't it love?' The Detective strolled in.

'Are you ready yet, darling?' he enquired of her.

'Are you having anything to eat, darling?' she replied, the diners still in a shocked, captivated state.

'Didn't I tell you I'm not hungry?'

With that, The Detective lifted his jacket from behind, shimmied his smooth arse at the horrified clientele and left arm in arm with his date. Minge looked behind her and laughed in contempt at the windowful of diners who were rubbing furiously at the condensation, craning for a last look at this strangest of couples, some of them presumably wondering whether alcohol and kebabs could act as an hallucinogen under certain clinical conditions. Minge had the last word.

'Bye bye my darlings!'

If The Detective had met his match in Minge then he was thoroughly enjoying every minute of it: their carnival of what the substance addiction treatment centres refer to as 'strange and insane behaviour' had only just begun as they headed back to the hotel for a night of awfulness between the sheets. The following morning Minge rang down to Reception and enquired what time the chamber maids came into the room. 'It's up to yourself, Missus,' came the standard reply. 'We can arrange it to suit your requirements. What time would be convenient for you?'

Half an hour later Minge and The Detective were ready to put on another grand show for yet another captive audience. She had opened all the doors and drawn back the curtains in the two rooms with the outside windows. They had pulled the bed underneath the biggest window in full view of several other rooms on the second floor.

When the chamber maids knocked at the unlocked door The Detective announced in his best policeman tones, 'come in Missus, the door's open.' 'Alright, love, cold morning isn't it?' said the slightly built middle-aged dear with the silver hair and regulation plastic overclothes as she slowly made her way in. A woman of similar age and dress pushing a trolley containing towels, soap and fresh bed linen, trundled in behind. Just then Minge and The Detective saddled up doggy style on the bed, as naked as Jay birds, and began their mad, ranting sex show. 'Oh my sacred heart of Je . . .,' one of the cleaners gulped as Minge roared like a hyena from the bed through the open window while the detective straddled her, huffing and puffing for all he was worth. The two chambermaids hadn't moved as quickly in fifty years.

Back on the road, the thrills were only just beginning as the clock struck midday. Both the rakish prostitute with the goatee red pubic hair and The Detective who found her so takish were completely naked as he drove through the city centre, up and down the capital's main thoroughfare of O'Connell Street twice before heading out to her brother's retail store not far from the city centre. By this time, a motorcyclist who had drawn up beside them and managed to see that their bottom halves were as exposed as the top couldn't resist tailing them as far as Thomas Street where his voyeurism got the better of him on a sharp bend. He went careering into the back of The Detective's car and his one-man mobile peek show came to a painful halt. What sort of statements he gave to the police and the insurance company regarding the lead-up to the accident is anyone's guess.

The incident provoked perhaps the one act of sanity this pair had experienced together in the past forty-eight hours when Minge decided not to call in and say hello to the brother, an image conscious and long suffering executive who had just about tired of trying to put his wayward sister on the straight and narrow and who by now must have been praying that she'd emigrate to Neptune. While sorely tempted to embarrass him even further, Minge ordered her driver to head for the hills instead. They had already planned to spend a night in the Dublin Mountains – the Hell Fire Club on Montpelier Hill, to be exact, a strange and remote place built by the Speaker Conolly in the early 1720s as a kind of eighteenth century rock and roll club for the blue bloods.

High in the hills with the tiny sparkling lights of the city dotted all around them as they surveyed the night-time vista from this long since disused building where the drunken loutish sons of the aristocracy met to perform rites of the occult among other nefarious acts of indulgence in their mad, mad parties of wickedness and sex – and where the Devil in cloven feet is said to have appeared during a card game, the Detective must have felt strangely at home. He went to the back of the car and took out his long black robe, his giant crucifix and his silver goblets. If the occasion was ever right for a woman to conceive his baby, Satan's baby, then tonight was the night . . .

The Detective took early retirement from the police a short time later and spent it out of Ireland. He has since died. While abroad, he wrote frequently to his soul mate Minge, imploring her to join him there. She didn't. She is now married to a former client of the Kasbah. She has several children, though none of them by Satan. She was working in various massage parlours up to the point when the Kasbah was raided in 1991. Like so many other 'masseuses' since that raid and the ensuing anti-brothel legislation she's back plying her trade on the streets.

Whatever fragile support systems were in place for Minge when she worked out of the brothels, they're gone now because her fear of being arrested has put her on the streets. This is thanks to a government which professed the desire to bring about a new beginning within conservative Ireland; an era of 'monuments of social change', to use Labour Party leader and Deputy Prime Minister Dick Spring's own words. What he and his colleague in the Justice Ministry have done, in fact, is to take away the one change in the working lives of prostitutes that offered some protection, some form of collectivity. The parlours were a *real* monument of change that had nothing to do with government-inspired philanthropy.

Chapter Thirteen

A Policeman's Lot . . .

Minge's naked jaunt through the streets of Dublin with The Detective provided fodder for conversation among the prostitutes of Dublin for months. Linda Lavelle was laughing, too, but this time her mirth was tempered by her fine-tuned grasp of reality: Minge was known in both police and vice circles as a Kasbah girl through and through and her recent spectacular adventures with The Detective, while appealing to the 'looper' which undoubtedly resides inside Linda herself, also concerned her that this sort of event would only serve to attract the wrong sort of police attention. She had learned the hard way that if you stayed within the limits of discretion and order, the authorities were not likely to give you any trouble, unless, of course, an official complaint was made which virtually compelled them to respond.

The Kasbah had only once found itself in the public eye in the six years of its existence when in 1987 the *Sunday World* newspaper's undercover journalists had exposed it as a brothel fronting as a health and fitness club. Many such parlours were exposed by the same newspaper during that period and the Kasbah was just one more: there was nothing to suggest that the girls who worked there were providing anything other than the usual strip massage, reverse massage, Swedish massage, hand relief, full sex, oral sex, and, of course, a straightforward massage. (For the record, Marion Murphy, the woman who was eventually charged with brothel-keeping at the Kasbah, is a qualified masseuse, having received her diploma from the Irish Health Culture Association on 15 April 1984.)

Because of the sheer number of brothels exposed by the newspaper, police reaction to it was relatively minimal. Privately, detectives who remembered the bloody street wars of the 1970s involving prostitutes and their pimps were more than happy to see the vice trade, or a substantial part of it, contained in premises away from public view, and there was certainly no moral objection to the brothels within the body of the force.

When complaints were lodged about a massage parlour known as the Galaxy Health Studio on 122 North Circular Road, Dublin, in the early weeks of 1984, however, the police had a double reason to act, and act fast. The brothel was being run by one of their own members, Garda Thomas Quinn and his wife Gloria, who both lived in the posh northside suburb of Laurel Lodge, Castleknock. A police estimate at the time put the cash turnover at the Galaxy in the region of £3,000 a week – not a bad sideline for a cop who was in line for a bravery award for coming to the aid of colleague Patrick Reynolds during a shoot-out at a house in the sprawling working-class suburb of Tallaght in February 1982. Had Quinn not drawn his baton in time, he would never have had to face the ignominy of court action which spelt personal and career disaster for him. For a bullet from the gun of one of Officer Reynolds' assailants split Quinn's baton in two as he lay beside his dying partner at the bottom of the blood-soaked stairs in a house in Avonbeg Gardens.

The court had to wait seven years before hearing another case involving brothel-keeping. This time it was the flamboyant and mercurial figure of Tom McDonnell who is said to be

£1 million better off as a result of his vice operations in Dublin. He was ordered to pay £4,500 to the Womens' Refuge Centre and narrowly avoided his old stomping ground of Mountjoy Jail when he was further sentenced to 100 hours of community service and a four-month suspended jail stint on sentences relating to the keeping of a brothel. The penalties handed down by Judge Michael Moriarty in the Dublin Circuit Court didn't worry McDonnell nearly as much as the fact that the Revenue Commissioners were on his tail for a share of his vice-propagated fortune.

The successful prosecution of Tom McDonnell marked a departure in police technique. For this first time, video surveillance was used to record the clients entering and leaving the bordello at Richmond Hill in Rathmines. On that occasion, police took the procedure one step further than in the later, celebrated raid on the Kasbah. The cameras actually went into McDonnell's brothel in the southside flatlands suburb and, in the classic 'police speak' of courtroom evidence, 'found a man naked and in a state of sexual arousal'. The man – a sailor – was being masturbated by a young masseuse. (He later said in court that he was being given treatment for an old sports injury!)

Former County Clare lorry driver McDonnell was seen in some quarters as an uncompromising and overly ambitious overlord within the Dublin vice world. Yet many of the prostitutes interviewed for this book felt that they had got a good deal from him. One of them – Vikki – told me, 'He was alright. Tom was alright. There was no messin' around, no funny business with Tom. If you did your side of things and got on with the job then he'd look after you okay. You could do a lot worse than Tom McDonnell.'

One woman not likely to share those sentiments, however, is former Kasbah prostitute Tanya, a slightly built middle-aged woman from working-class Dublin, known also to her colleagues for some obscure reason as How's Your Father.

Tanya's one persistent drawback to the smooth running of her day was her eyesight: she had very little of it. Linda Lavelle remembers, 'When a client would knock at the door, Tanya would head straight to the room for her glasses and put them on. She'd take them off again as soon as she opened the door and before the caller would see her because she felt they were a turn-off for the client. She was fucking right!'

Once, while working for McDonnell, Tanya was experiencing the commonplace difficulty of locating her spectacles or her contact lenses. She was literally tumbling around the walls of a brothel in Capel Street looking for them when a knock came at the door. She told her boss McDonnell that she couldn't answer the door without her seeing aids and the short-tempered West of Ireland man lost his reason. Said Linda, 'One of Tom McDonnell's associates, male associates, was coming at her with an axe or something. At least that's what Tanya thought. It was probably one of the men having a roar at her, that's all. She couldn't have known because she was so fucking blind, but she made her way to the front door and ran out the place as quick as she could.'

People who believe their lives to be in imminent danger are apt to take a single-minded course of action with scant regard for the rituals of civilised behaviour. And so it was with How's Your Father as she ran almost the length of a busy shopping street on a Saturday morning wearing a white basque and a quite terrified expression. Visually unaided, she collided with at least two cars as she headed for a safe-house – another massage parlour a couple of hundred yards away – in her frenzied escape from a man who wasn't even following her, although it would have been impossible for her to know that as she looked around at the sea of blurred figures on the pavements. Tanya survived relatively unscathed, which is more than can be said for at least one bus which ran into the back of a parked car during her ricochet run through the traffic. Settled and visually equipped again, Tanya was until recently running a brothel known as Rosebud in Protestant Row off Wexford Street, its main claim to fame being a Discipline dungeon operated by her and a buxom blonde with the unlikely title of Madame Germaine.

Tanya is remembered fondly, but with sarcasm, by the Kasbah girls for one oddity among her many oddities. Said Linda, 'She had this really odd habit of announcing to everyone "the gentleman is now leaving" when she'd be finished with a client and he was heading to the door. We all joined in the skit by waving our hands and saying together, "Bye bye, all the best, now" to the mortified poor man whoever he was.'

In the 1980s, sporadic trouble, particularly in the so-called 'meat beat' zones was still erupting. On 29 May 1985, four women, two of them self-confessed prostitutes, were deported from Ireland after vicious faction-fighting erupted among the streetwalkers of Fitzwilliam Square involving the girls from England and local women. In one such attack, King's Cross prostitute Shirley Bronn was set upon in her flat in Rathmines by girls wielding iron bars and flick-knives in a row over £200 in takings they claimed she had stolen from them.

The attack had little to do with the money, however. The four deportees had already planned a speedy exit from Ireland after being warned by Irish prostitutes in Fitzwilliam Square that there would be real trouble in store for them that weekend if they didn't clear off back to England. The Bronn incident was just 'unfinished business': the women had already purchased their tickets for the Dún Laoghaire–Holyhead ferry earlier that day.

Five years later the prostitutes of Dublin would be given a grim reminder of just how inherently dangerous street life was, both in the form of internecine struggles, and sometimes the clients themselves. It arrived in the form of a chronic alcoholic named Patrick Barr, a thirty-five-year-old father of three who performed unspeakable atrocities with a stick on a twenty-two-year-old prostitute after picking her up in his white van on Fitzwilliam Square and driving her to the Phoenix Park a couple of miles away. Afterwards, he dumped her on a back road. The four crinkled up £5 notes he had handed over to the woman who had given birth only two weeks earlier had nearly cost her her life on that balmy July night of 1991.

Barr returned to the Fitzwilliam Square meat-beat four weeks later to pick up another girl and, presumably, assault her as well. His white van was an easy giveaway for the two young detectives, Philip Ryan and Terry Kenny, who had lain in wait for weeks in the hope of spotting the man who told his victim that he was the Devil. Before he committed his gross acts of buggery and assault on the terrified young prostitute, Barr boasted to her of how he murdered two women and buried their bodies. The depravity of his actions and his rantings about what he did with women or what he'd wish to do with them, may have had more to do with the stage of his addiction to booze than anything else, although that was cold comfort to the women walking the streets at night.

The Barr episode was different in one fundamental regard to general trade in the massage parlours, particularly the Kasbah, where the prostitutes also participated in the most atrocious sexual encounters with their male clients: at the bordello the women knew what they were buying into and they could choose and refuse their clients – they had that choice and they had some form of protection to back it up.

The question of whether men like Patrick Barr, whose depravities (alcohol-triggered or not) led to so much suffering and unrecorded humiliation in the female population, could be rendered less dangerous by allowing them to live out that otherwise inhibited part of their lives with women who are to some degree prepared for it and paid handsome sums for it is one that could be debated for a long time without any clear answers emerging.

Would the Patrick Barrs of this world become even more

insatiable, volatile and extreme in their behaviour, by being exposed to this kind of à la carte perversion whenever something snapped in their minds compelling them to satisfy their awful needs?

The emergence of the massage parlours in Dublin had, it seemed, once and for all broken the organised grip of the pimps and dramatically lessened the dangers for the women working in prostitution in Dublin. A decade after the street wars it was the women prostitutes themselves who controlled the vice business. There were pimps, of course, but their influence and power was largely reserved for the 'one-man' operations involving a prostitute working the streets for the man she was living with and propping up financially.

'What is a pimp?' asks Linda Lavelle. 'I suppose a boyfriend or a husband of a girl on the game is a pimp just as much as the guy who sends two or three girls out on the streets and collects the readies off them in return for some form of protection that they don't really need anymore. Pimps come in many guises, pimps do. But they're not all dangerous.

'Not any more.'

Chapter Fourteen

'To Have And To Hold . . .'

Demand among a particular section of the Irish public for the exquisite excesses of the Kasbah's brand of sex was such that by 1986 the prostitutes working there had achieved the hitherto undreamt of luxury of picking and choosing their clients. On busy days, and most of the days were extremely busy, punters would be asked at the door if they were clients of other massage parlours in the area and if it transpired that the Kasbah was their alternative choice they would be simply turned away. 'They just weren't worth it,' explained Pia. 'We had more business than we could handle as things stood.'

Uniquely, the Kasbah had also become a meeting place for prostitutes – a working girls' club as one of them described it – who plied the inner city on both sides of the river. They would regularly drop in to the Kasbah for mid-morning coffee beside the omnipresent coal fire. (The fire blazed even on the hottest summer days, its main function was not to keep the girls cosy so much as to destroy evidence such as used condoms and sex aids in the event of a police raid.)

It wasn't unusual, for instance, to see young children in the basement of 60B Mountjoy Square West, particularly on special Church occasions such as confirmations and First Holy Communions. Prostitutes from all round the city would take their children on the traditional day-long visit to friends and relations who would often include their working mates at the Kasbah. And clients would sometimes give the children money as they sat around playing on the floor while their mothers gaggled away smoking cigarettes and drinking tea on the sofa, the conversation dividing equally between the cost of the kids' clothes for the day and gossip surrounding clients. What the Catholic hierarchy would have made of such visits as part of the process of these important spiritual events in the calendar of their Church can only be imagined.

The occasion of the wedding of Joanne Kelly's sister, Lorraine (not her real name), was one of supreme irony and not a little confusion for the men and women of the Kasbah. For several weeks prior to the big day, a little old lady called Dolly (not her real name) would arrive at the basement looking for prostitutes with requisite bust, hip, waist and leg measurements, etc., to try out the white silk dress she was so painstakingly putting together. Regulars among the steady stream of clients thought it was just another little earner for Linda, some scam or other in a world of scams and double-bluff and fantasy; or maybe she was executing a good deed for someone in need. Everyone, including the clients, knew that Linda could be both motherly and charitable as well as rapier sharp, sometimes moving from one to another at a stroke.

On the day before the wedding the dress was laid out in all its glory on the striped sofa along with the dresses for the bridesmaids, the bouquets of flowers, white patent shoes, etc. The thirty or so clients who passed through the doors of the Kasbah that day all reacted differently, Linda recalls. 'Some of them were asking me which one of the girls was getting married! One man dug deep into his pocket to give a money gift. Others were fearful that one of their favourite girls was getting married and they wouldn't be able to screw her or whatever anymore. That worried a lot of them.'

They need not have been unduly concerned, for the woman

destined for her nuptials was a respectable middle-class medic. The fact that she had once worked as a prostitute in the Kasbah for six months in order to finance her honeymoon to the other side of the planet with her lovestruck and unemployed paramour was of passing interest to her former work mates and clients alike as old Dolly began sewing the fake pearl buttons onto the lily-white dress.

The fact that the work had been designated to Dolly was a nice touch. The seamstress who lent so much moral support to Linda and the other prostitutes during the Kasbah trial in 1993 was herself a former prostitute who, at fifty-six years of age, could no longer demand a proper fee from clients – except, of course, from the deviants with a fetish for granny types – and she was quite destitute: like so many of her contemporaries in the vice game, the big bucks came and the big bucks went; life was lived for today and when tomorrow finally arrived no one quite knew what to do about it. There are hundreds of Dollys in Dublin alone, ex-prostitutes now broken, bitter, bemused and worn out with little other than State welfare to see them through until they meet their Maker. There are only a few Linda Lavelles: women who make prostitution work for them, who manage to manipulate it before it takes hold of their soul and fries them up with self-loathing, drug or alcohol addiction and, eventually, leaves them in much the same way it found them, only older and less able to cope.

Up to six women would work each daily cycle at the Kasbah, dividing shifts into day time (11am to 5pm) and night time (5pm to 10.30pm). Linda Lavelle was always the *grande Madam*, even when Poppy Healy thought *she* was the boss, taking in £15 book money from the clients who would sometimes number forty a day, seven days a week.

By this stage Linda had built a magnificent five-bedroomed detached home in a posh suburb on the northside of Dublin and still had plenty of money left over in the bank. With clients being turned away at the Kasbah and with a list of girls queueing up to work there as prostitutes, the time had come for expansion. On 14 June 1986 she opened a second brothel known as Laura's Studio in nearby Belvedere Place which was run like a branch office of the Kasbah, the girls taking shifts at both bordellos but the favoured ones remaining inside the lucrative and shocking walls of 60B Mountjoy Square West.

Laura's never quite reached the dizzy depths of perversion and depravity enjoyed by so many at the Kasbah – although it promised much when the premises were 'officially' opened by a client known as the Rubber Back Carpet Man, a well known, respected and wealthy figure within the world of Irish industry (who had no connection with floor coverings!), whose expertise in laying carpets was never quite matched by his enthusiasm or speed. As a gift to the girls, the R.B.C.M. presented them with the highest quality carpet and underlay that money could buy for their newly acquired and more spacious premises. The quality of the merchandise was assured only by the price he paid for it as the man had little or no knowledge of carpets.

One evening at around 10pm he delivered his gift to 24 Belvedere Place. If he was expecting appreciation he had made an error of judgement. Pia surveyed the long rolls of green, pink and blue carpet and underlay being brought in from the van outside and piled up in the hall.

'What the fuck are we going to do with this for Jesus' sake? What are you going to do with all of this? You can't leave it here. We have a fucking business to run and this shit is getting in the way.'

Eight hours later, according to Pia and other prostitutes, the job was done and the R.B.C.M. was at least a stone lighter, having single-handedly lain all the underlay and carpets in three rooms, a hall and on the stairs, all the while wearing a rubber diving suit he had squashed himself into before his arrival that day. For this client was a Slave and as such would do whatever was asked of him while in role. Had Pia shown more appropriate appreciation for his donation she would have betrayed his fantasy of being treated like dirt by a woman. His favourite fetish was dressing up in tight-fitting leather or rubber that he would purchase on his frequent trips to England and Europe. He supplied his own box of talcum powder each time he visited the girls: an essential requirement for getting out of the skin-tight suits once his session was complete.

The night after he had put down the carpets, the Rubber Back Carpet Man was back in Laura's, this time with a hamper, to continue his bizarre opening celebrations. A grand buffet was served in the front room overlooking the street outside. Girls on the Kasbah shift arrived for the party and the champagne and vodka flowed into the early hours thanks to the strange and secret mind of another family man who to this day is at the heart of Irish commercial life.

But fine carpets and vintage champagne do not make a crazy sex-rub joint and the exquisitely brothel-ly atmosphere in the Kasbah was never fully achieved in the bordello on Belvedere Place. (The entire house at number 24 was eventually sold off in July 1994.) For one thing, the rooms were too big and airy. Linda and the girls couldn't make a Kasbah Mark II out of it, no matter how sinfully hard they tried.

Linda said, 'Laura's was very successful but it never had that thing that the Kasbah possessed. I don't know what it is. It never seemed to attract the real nutters, the specialist clients, in the same way. A lot of men went into Laura's just for straight sex and in that sense it suited a lot of the girls. But from a professional point of view, our profession, it was never as fulfilling a place as the Kasbah. It was never as exciting or brothel-ly. And it was never as busy as the Kasbah. Jesus, there were times you couldn't get into that place. But Laura's always had its quiet times for the girls where they could take life a lot easier.'

Whatever else may be said about her as a person and as a madam to a brothel, Linda Lavelle's expertise and love for her chosen lifestyle is what really marks her out. By all accounts, she is supremely accomplished at her work. One suspects that her natural talents would have brought her to the pinnacle of whatever line of work she had entered but such alternatives were, it seems, never near her thoughts. 'I would never have wanted to work at anything else from the minute I got into this game. Every client is different – even the Discipline clients. It's not all about hitting and caning mens' legs and bottoms . . . and in a sense you get a certain buzz out of every client you look after because each of them is so different. I'd much prefer doing something like that than working in a grotty office or a bank where each day tumbles into the next and each day is the same.'

Mandy Jameson adds, 'Most men have a kink in one way or the other and that's why they'd come to us in the first place; they wouldn't dare tell their wives or partners about [their fantasies] so they use us to play out whatever part they wanted. I don't feel one bit bad about that. I was a married woman and I prostituted myself for en suite showers and fucking dishwashers and new clothes. At least I'm doing it now with a bit more honesty and most of the time I'm generally doing it with men I'm happy enough to be with sexually so don't give me any of that crap about not being respectable. Everyone prostitutes themselves in one form or another.'

While straight sex, hand relief, strip massage, Swedish massage, reverse relief have set prices, such services were never really part of the mainstream scene at the Kasbah. 'The men with the perversions,' said Kasbah girl Pia, 'would pay anything you want. They would pay us literally anything. Last Tuesday, for instance, I got a call from some man over on the southside. I had to go to his house but when I pulled up outside the place he was hanging out the window and beckoning me to go on up the road. I thought, "this is a bummer", but two minutes later he comes over to my car and said his father and brother had come back unexpectedly so I couldn't go in as planned. He told me there was no trouble in paying me and asked me to wait. A few minutes later he arrived back again and this time got into the car and he said he just wanted to talk to me. We drove to a pub and had an orange juice. He told me he was after being in a car accident and had received a lot of money.

'I arranged to meet him the following day at his home at the same time. I got £500 off him just to drive him around Dublin telling him that his mother was only a whore. He kept feeding me with what he wanted to hear me say. He wanted to get the mother put into a room and have ten lesbians thrown in on top of her. He kept saying that he saw his mother in the nude a few times and that he would love to rape her. He said he would love to see his father being raped by a black man. This went on for about an hour and a half. He was twenty-seven years old. People would be horrified if they knew who he was. He managed to spend on me a total of £650 in about two hours. He had this thing about homosexuals and kept asking me did he know any gay men. He asked whether he could work for me for nothing. He wasn't homosexual himself – no way – but he had a real fixation about them. He kept assuring me that money was no object and that he wanted a girl to rip him off. I mean, it was weird. He loves women to fucking rip him off; he kept telling me, "please, Pia, rip me off. Here, take my money."'

Pia obliged. She received several thousand pounds from this particular client before she was finished. 'It was easy money.'

There was nothing easy, however, about meeting the requirements of another regular client known to the Kasbah women only as Mister Half Head. His patronage is poignantly sad in its broken-spirited despair. Said Linda, 'All the girls used to hate Mister Half Head coming into the place. They used to be saying to me, "I can't do that man anymore, don't give him to me, Linda."'

Mister Half Head was suffering from cancer. One side of his face had been eaten away by the disease with just mottled red scar tissue in its place. He knew the girls hated doing him, not that there was any physical sexual content to his terms. It was actually much worse than that for the women, much more difficult to handle. Explained Linda, 'He'd come in and ask for some slow music to be put on. Then he'd hold one of the girls in a slow dance for half an hour. That was it. Jesus Christ it was horrible but what do you say to such a poor bastard as him? "Sorry, we can't do you, we refuse to do you. We can't fucking stand to be near you now fuck off out of here?" Imagine how he'd feel if he was barred from a brothel? Life was shit enough for him without being barred from a brothel.'

For exactly half an hour but for what must have seemed like half a lifetime, Mister Half Head slowly danced, his destroyed face resting gently on the shoulder of his serving woman. They played tunes, his tunes – Acker Bilk's *Stranger on the Shore* and Andy Williams's *Moon River* – in one of the tiny dimly lit rooms with the red glow-bulb. Not a word would ever be spoken as the music droned on, not a tear shed, in this deafeningly sad statement of one man's isolation and his hired woman's reluctant, but never once denied, succour.

Mister Half Head has since passed away. I couldn't help guessing, as the prostitutes told me his story on several occasions, that he had been nourished in some way or other during his visits to the Kasbah. Nor could I help thinking of how difficult it had been for the women of the brothel to tell this story, a story of their soulful concern for another human being as they dressed their charity – as usual – in brittle scorn.

It was a complete change – and a refreshing one – for the girls to engage a dashingly handsome and well-known Northern Ireland businessman who went under the cheeky but apt name of Northern Dick. 'One day he came down and brought this fucking thing with him, a strap-a-dick-to-me,' said Mandy Jameson. 'Myself and another girl, Susan, were doing him when he produced this dick and said that he wanted to be raped, fucked with the rubber dick. For ten minutes she [Susan] rammed this fucking thing into his arse while he wanked himself off. The whole idea was that he wanted to be raped by a man. He would have been far happier if there had been a few gay men around the place.'

Placed pretty well on the same wacky wavelength to Dick, was a high-ranking civil servant from County Cork with the far less flattering title of Cork Shithead. Linda explained, 'He got the same sort of service as Northern Dick but after every session he would go in for a shower and crap in one of the towels and leave it there. I think it's some form of buried aggression.'

No week at the Kasbah would be complete without a visit from a professional man self-styled as Maid Maggie. Like Dick and Cork Shithead, he would arrive at the Kasbah carrying his bag of tricks and head straight for one of the custom built cubicles. Less than five minutes later he would come out wearing an old blue floral apron and an oil-stained countryman's cloth cap. His get-up was signal enough for the girls who would immediately start shouting the chorus, 'Maid Maggie, Maid Maggie, has anyone seen Maid Maggie?' while they ran around the place in theatrical search.

Up to that point his fantasy seemed, well, almost normal, but it would not stay that way for very long. Explained Susan, 'His kink was to arrive at a gypsy camp with all the men and women standing around a fire. He would join the men in talk but as soon as they were gone off on their rounds he would mix in with the gypsy women and start riding all the gypsy women. He would visualise that he'd be riding all the women in the Phoenix Park or out in a field somewhere or sometimes in a hayshed . . . never in a bed. He'd be ranting on about their big wide dresses and their big gypsy knickers and how he'd lift one up and pull the other down. The Maid Maggie bit was part of the fantasy where he'd have fooled the gypsy menfolk into thinking that he was one of the women maids and he'd only reveal himself as a man as soon as they're all gone off for the day.'

The Irish legal community was not found wanting in its provision of a regular and plentiful crop of clients to the Kasbah over its ten years of trade. And 'crop' is not a bad word to use in relation to many of them. Explained Linda Lavelle, 'Generally speaking they are a simple enough bunch to handle. Nearly all of them were into various forms of Discipline which meant that I got to know a lot of them personally. One gentleman in particular – the whole country knows this fellow – loves to strip naked and get into a pair of high-heels and black fishnet stockings and have me whip the back of his legs off with a cane until he jerks off. Another gentleman, a solicitor, was into the same sort of thing although he didn't care for the stockings. I know people will find all this hard to believe. I only mention these two men because they are so public. People would be really shocked if they knew the sort of names who used to come into the Kasbah for their sex and for Discipline.'

Another client, a well-known and respected figure in Irish broadcasting, had a relationship with his own semen which proved too much for Charlene Robertson. 'He started off pretty okay. He'd come in looking for a massage and he'd often have full sex and there was really nothing that kinky about him at all. Then one night he asked me whether I'd mind getting a cup for him so that he could drink his cum after sex. I told him no problem. I didn't really believe him because a lot of men say things like that but they never do it. Next thing I saw him put the cup beside him as I was getting dressed after sex and the fucker was emptying his condom into it. I thought to myself, "Suffering Jesus, get out of here, he's going to do it" and I made sure my back was turned to him. The next thing he said was, "Li-iz, oh Li-iz" [he always called her Liz] and like an eejit I turned around and he knocked it back. I vomited right there as I was running out of the room. But that was his kink – to see the girl getting sick. That's what it was all about for him. It wasn't about swallowing his own spunk; it was about seeing me throw up. Another time he caught me off guard when he didn't ask for the cup. Then he called my name again as he was getting out of the shower after sex. I turned around and there he was sucking out the contents of his condom. I threw up again. He was a sadistic bastard.'

The broadcasting man, known to girls as Cup of Cum among other dreadful nicknames, was also unpredictably violent. He is one of the few clients that the prostitutes felt physically threatened by.

Linda would always look for two of her most seasoned girls when she received a phone call from a man living in a posh southside suburb who, unbeknown to himself to this day, had been given the intriguing name of The Undertaker. 'He became a two-girl client from the time he gave up kerb-crawling in the late 1970s,' she recalled. 'He lives alone as far as anyone of us could make out and when the girls would call out to his house he would have a full-sized coffin laid out in the sitting room!'

The Undertaker may have been an eerie sort of customer, but the girls loved looking after him. It was pure theatre, and, despite the coffin and the other morbid accessories, there was never any indication that he was either dangerous or satanic. One of the girls, very often Vikki, would have to get into the box, undressed, and covered by a white mortuary shroud, with her hands entwined in rosary beads and folded in the rite of the dead. The other girl, often Linda, would be presented with a bunch of freshly cut flowers by The Undertaker (his actual job couldn't be further removed from that of a mortician) and she would walk around the coffin mumbling prayers and sprinkling holy water on top of the 'corpse', as per instructions. The

Undertaker would just sit there. Inscrutable. Watching. Staring at the girl as she delivered her mantras over a hooker in a wooden box who was barely able to contain herself. Then, as the boxing commentators are fond of putting it, things started to hot up after the opening round. Said Linda, 'He'd just take off all his clothes and start following the girl around the coffin wanking himself and shouting "Fuck you Josephine for dying, fuck you Josephine for dying."'

It's not surprising that the girls at the Kasbah liked to finish their shift in a pub: a girl needs to unwind after playing host to an undertaker, a monkey, or whatever other strange cases the world was constantly throwing at their feet. It was also very serious work, too. Staying in role required tremendous self-control and was a prerequisite to the success of the service they were providing. Said Linda Lavelle, 'The girls always laughed about what the clients got up to. They were always having a good fucking giggle at what the men required them to do. I suppose it relieved the tension of the work. But they could never laugh *at* the client: something like that just isn't on. No professional woman would ever laugh at a client. It would be disastrous if clients even *thought* that we were having fun at their expense.'

The most unlikely venues were often chosen by the women to let off steam for an hour: the Tudor Rooms in nearby Barry's Hotel close to the Kasbah, the hotel's own bastion of traditional conservative values, was a case in point. The hotel was and is run as a bona fide piece of rural heartland based in the middle of the city. On many nights there was dancing in the Tudor Rooms, to the sounds of traditional Irish or country and western music. It was in these rooms that scores of displaced lonely and mostly middle-aged hearts originally from the provinces would flock in the dark hours, yearning to taste again the scents of love and romance and perhaps a bit of passion.

Business permitting, the girls at the Kasbah would switch

off the lights and lock the front steel door in time for a tipple or two in Barry's before making their separate ways home. It was a practice that did not go unnoticed by their clientele who often stopped off at the hotel if they arrived at the Kasbah to find that the tell-tale glow from behind the heavy curtain over the basement window had been prematurely extinguished and trade had closed for the day. Despite the public perception, massage parlour women and other prostitutes don't actually *look* any different to other women once out of their working gear, with the possible exception of Vikki who appeared to devote a considerable portion of her life living up to her own image as that of a 'total whore'. So when the girls hit the Tudor Rooms in Barry's they looked like so many other women there: in search of company. In search of a man . . .

Explained Linda, 'We'd sit up at the bar and have a few drinks and get into conversation. But I suppose the real entertainment was looking at these women dancing with the men. Some of these men were regular clients of ours and that used to give us a right fucking laugh. The women would be thinking what a fine catch they had in this fella or that and he'd be on his best behaviour, full of manners and oul charm. What the women didn't know was that a few of them were Kasbah clients and they had come to the hotel looking for us! They were only dancing with the women because they were nervous about coming over to us in public. A lot of them were out and out fucking perverts and they had no interest in the women they were dancing with. If Mandy was with us she'd catcall over at them while they were dancing with the ladies. She'd say, "Hey Jim, or hey Joe, or Paddy, will you be alright for a bit later you old fart!" and things like that. It was a right mad scream.'

It goes without saying that the staff at this well-run hotel couldn't possibly have had any idea of the furtive goings-on of the Kasbah girls in their midst.

Chapter Fifteen

Profiles In Atrocity

When a well-known actor turned down a film role which required him to strip naked for a bedroom scene, observers of the film world expressed their disapproval at his decision – but not surprise. He had no trouble arguing that a nude scene – even for a male – was not a good career move. The movie in question was not his kind of thing anyway, he said, and he really wanted to work on the stage – a pretentious and egotistical explanation so often adopted, and condoned, in his line of work.

What none of his audience could have known, however, was that to have taken the nude film part would have exposed his other life as a sex Slave to vice women from all over Europe. For this actor carried branding marks on his buttocks from brothels in Amsterdam, England, and, of course, from the Kasbah. Branding is used to enforce a kind of status order among clients of brothels. It is a much sought after accolade because not every Madam is prepared to go through with the ritual of depressing a red-hot trade mark into the behind of one of her men. The letter 'K' had long since been burned deep into the actor's flesh, an outward testimony to his inner sexual self: his hired women, and his quite awful mores. For he was no ordinary client – if that term can ever be appositely used in connection with the business of paid vice, particularly in the Kasbah. He wasn't even an ordinary deviant in the sense of being satisfied by kink, fantasy or downright odd behaviour. For the actor, known to all the girls in the Kasbah as Smelly Bottoms, was a student of perhaps the most odious and, for me at least, stomach-churning form of abnormal behaviour: its clinical name is scatology, defined in the dictionary as obscene interest in human excrement. He was one of many such clients to use the Kasbah and, as Linda Lavelle points out, virtually all such men were 'own bosses' types, 'People who were looked up to in their work and who everyone else in the job tried to copy.'

Like all Slaves, Smelly Bottoms was at the mercy of the Kasbah women while in role: and they were merciless to him as to no other client. During his weekly sessions, the prostitutes would take him to the surrounding pubs at his behest. In one alehouse not far from the brothel and where some of the girls were known to the staff, Smelly Bottoms was once brought in and told by Mandy to sit in a corner and behave himself. 'He was wearing a big long coat and a pair of black tights which were full of his own shite,' she recalls. 'Me and Vikki just put him sitting in the corner and told him to buy us drink and be good and fucking quiet for the next few hours.' And that's exactly what this strangest of men did, not appearing to notice the steady stream of drinkers who changed their seating positions to be as far away from him as possible.

Said Mandy, 'Every twenty minutes or so I would saunter over to him and say, "Get your mistress another drink and hurry up about it or I'll take it out now and you know what that means, don't you?"' She would open her black handbag and give him a peek at the coiled six-foot long black leather whip inside and Smelly Bottoms would reply, 'You wouldn't use that on me, Mistress Mandy. You wouldn't use that on me in here would you, not where everyone knows you, not where all your friends are?' Mandy's riposte was, as usual, full of menace. 'Don't bet on it. Don't bet on it, you dirty little smelly horrible bastard. One more word of cheek out of you and I'll take this whip out and whip you right outside the door of this pub in front of everyone right the way back down to the Kasbah where you belong.'

How much of this invective was based on Mandy's true feelings and how much of it was commissioned farce for the £200 Smelly Bottoms had given her earlier, is difficult to tell. The drinkers in the pub that night found the whole business very odd. One of them remarked, 'You'd think he'd stand up to her. I wouldn't take that sort of thing from a woman. Not if she was the fucking Queen.' Even the barman who had seen Mandy bring in some oddballs in his time, was intrigued. 'Who's that lamp in the corner sending you over drink all night, Mandy?' to which she replied, 'You wouldn't believe it if I told you what he's got underneath that coat he's wearing.'

The money the actor had paid earlier in the night and which had long since been spent by Mandy settling an overdue bill, was for a session in the Kasbah after closing time: the business in the pub was just a planned warm-up session. He didn't know it at the time, but his mistress had knocked back a few too many brandies and her favourite vodka and lemonades (bought by him) to consider working in the brothel for a while. Anyway, on this occasion she just couldn't stomach the thought of what he was really after that night: to be fed his own faeces with matchsticks.

Said Mandy, 'That just wasn't on that night. And he wasn't getting his money back, either. I said to myself that I'd make it up to him some other time.' Smelly Bottoms got something of a consolation in Discipline on that occasion, although he neither expected nor asked for it. As the tipplers filed out of the pub at closing time, Mandy walked over to him, unfurled the big black whip with an expert crack and hounded the awful-smelling and terrified actor/client out through the front doors with her drink-slurred remonstrations.

'Geddupowadat, you dirty, miserable, smelly little fucking

git. Take that, you smelly bastard. Take that out of the fucking fee.'

Smelly Bottoms disappeared into the night air. Very quickly.
Mandy made her way back into the pub, breathless from her
exertions. The phone rang. It was Margaret 'Poppy' Healy
who was stationed in the Kasbah waiting to receive Mandy
and her client as prearranged.

'Mandy, is that you? When are you coming down with the
client? I'm here all night. You can't keep the client waiting. It's
just not fair. Mandy, can you hear me? Answer me, will ya?'

'Fuck off, Poppy.'

That there were two distinct types inside the head of Smelly
Bottoms is undeniable. The man, who on another occasion
dressed in an open woman's coat, hat and black tights filled
with his own excrement and, as a Slave, walked into a crowded
fish and chip shop in broad daylight to collect sustenance for
the ladies of the Kasbah was also a deeply caring individual
whose work for charities was and still is enormous. He helped
out one of Linda Lavelle's sons when he was preparing a curriculum vitae and after the Kasbah court case in 1993 he called
around to the luxurious Lavelle household to express his com-
miseration, although that deed showed little insight into
Linda's need at that low point in her life which was to be at
home with her family and far away from the sort of pressures
he represented.

She remembers, 'He knocked on the door a few times and I
opened one of the top bedroom windows. He said he'd read
about the court case and wondered if there was anything he
could do to help. Jesus, I thought, the Kasbah's name and
address and photograph were in the papers that day along with
Marion Murphy and now Smelly Bottoms comes around to
my house. I shouted down to him, "Get the fuck out of here,
Smelly. I'm fit to jump out of this window, I'm feeling so low.
Get the fuck out of here."' Smelly Bottoms replied, 'You're in
need of a very good massage, Linda. And I'm just the man to

give it to you. And after that I will cook for you tonight. I do a very good curry.'

Of all the good and charitable deeds he was capable of performing, Linda Lavelle knew too much about Smelly Bottoms to contemplate eating one of his gastronomic creations. Particularly, she thought, a curry.

A disposition towards scatology was by no means the sole preserve of the man they called Smelly Bottoms, although he raised this practice to uniquely appalling levels at times. Linda recalls, 'Powerful people are into shit and piss and that kind of thing. We had one man who came in once a month for what he called his reward. He would bring in a china plate and asked one of the girls, usually Susan, for a nice hot meal.' Another businessman – he has literally hundreds of people working for him around the country – once presented Linda with a pair of Waterford Crystal goblets.

'At first I thought they were a gift to me but then I realised that they were part of his kink as a Slave. Every couple of weeks he would ask for his reward, he called it Madam's Champagne. We would put our champagne into the glasses and sit him at a table. He'd asked to be stripped naked and we'd tie him up in chains. He'd say, "It's beautiful, Madam, really beautiful. Don't worry, I won't spill any of it." His name was Sally and we would goad him, "Drink it slowly, Sally. You can't rush a fine drink like champagne. And if I catch any of it dribbling down your chin I'll whip you, you naughty boy." Imagine, this fucker was drinking our piss! Who could imagine a nutter like this coming into the Kasbah and complimenting the prostitutes on their piss, the piss he was drinking and an hour later he'd be back in his office with people jumping out of their seats to salute him.'

Linda Lavelle continued, 'But they [Slaves and fetish types] needed this service that we offered where they became nothings, where we made them into dogsbodies. These type of men went to the Kasbah and paid for that type of service because they required it, they wanted it. And they haven't changed just because the Kasbah's gone. They're still out there. Specialist clients will always be clients. No matter what society thinks, these men feel they are in need of the service that the girls at the Kasbah provided and they're not now just going to go away or reform themselves.' She added, 'Specialist clients like Smelly Bottoms will make more frequent visits to the stink chambers in Amsterdam now that the Kasbah's closed because the street girls in this country are not able to look after their needs properly. They have to get better, more professional at their professions, they have to get more used to it, before handling the likes of Smelly Bottoms.'

If these episodes of perversion and deviance on an unspeakably foul scale were part and parcel of the lives of the women at the Kasbah at least they were balanced to some extent by episodes of immense hilarity, like the day the building next door to the nondescript five storey Georgian building which housed the brothel became the focal point of national newspaper and television attention.

The Saturday morning had started off like most at the Kasbah: busy. Mandy, Vikki O'Toole and Charlene Robertson were on duty and had opened up at the usual time of 10.30am. Mandy more than the others was anxious to 'look after' a client as soon as possible: it was her daughter's birthday and she had ordered an inscribed cake for £15 from a nearby confectioners which was to be collected and paid for by noon when she planned to leave work early and start the festivities for the children in that other world of hers, the world of suburban, respectable motherhood.

The proceedings in the basement were rudely interrupted by the sounds of smashing glass on the pavement just outside the front window. Pots of paint, framed pictures and more glass rained down in a cacophony of mayhem as the three women strained at the window to get a look at what was going on. Above, they could hear a man and a woman shouting at each other as the debris continued to fall out of the sky. A brown car parked outside the railings had, in the blink of an eye, turned a glistening white. Traffic had ground to a halt and the entire street was cordoned off. Photographers were everywhere along with police cars, film crews, reporters, ambulances and fire fighters.

Suddenly a loud knock came on the black steel door of the Kasbah. A large policeman stood in front of Charlene, the glass still crunching under his shiny black boots. 'Is there any way through to the top? Is there any way up from here?' Mandy had answers to questions like that and it was perhaps fortunate that she didn't answer the door on this occasion. Charlene said, 'No. What's going on?' as Vikki headed straight to the toilet on hearing the knock, consigning her recreational pharmaceuticals to the city's sewage system . . . there would be a few happy rats down there that Saturday night. 'Fuck the rats and fuck the fuzz', she said.

Saturday is a traditionally slow news day in the Irish capital. To have what appeared to be an attempted suicide drama unfold in the city centre in time for the first editions of the two evening newspapers was greeted like manna from Heaven in the respective news rooms of the *Evening Herald* and its rival, the *Evening Press*. On the sub-editors' desk the lay-out men were already feverishly scribbling 'poss heads', (insider shorthand for possible headlines) as they tried to second-guess the intentions of the man standing on the gutter of the five-storey building unloading his artistic inventory on the unsuspecting Dublin public. 'DEATH JUMP IN CITY – Police talk-down mercy bid fails', or, in the equally newsworthy event of him maintaining his existence, 'COP HERO IN CITY SUICIDE DRAMA – "I'll jump" man talked down.'

So far the police had established that the man's name was Padraig, and that he was an artist, who lived next door to the Kasbah in 59 Mountjoy Square West and who had just had a row with his girlfriend.

'ARTIST IN CITY DEATH JUMP – Row with girlfriend ends in tragedy'. The three headlines were put aside in readiness to couple-up with the facts as they unfolded. What none of the hacks could have known, of course, was that the real news was below, and not above, the heads of the medical and security crews, as Vikki and a client well-known to the public humped for all they were worth in one of the little rooms off the dimly lit hallway only feet away from the prying eyes of the national press corps.

Padraig the artist had been a friend of Linda Lavelle's from the day the Kasbah opened in 1981, although in all the time he had known Linda and the other prostitutes he had not once expressed a sexual interest in any of them, executing his own life plan of live and let live. He had advised Linda on decor and presented her with a few tastefully erotic pictures which helped enormously with the atmosphere in the Kasbah. Once he had come up with a plan to get publicity for the bordello in the early days by suggesting that one of the girls go to the All Ireland hurling final later that year and streak across the pitch just before the starting whistle blew. He promised he'd paint the letters K.A.S.B.A.H on her back with the telephone number inscribed underneath. Both of them agreed that Vikki was the right woman for the job. Vikki, as ever, was game, too. Luckily for the stout souls who make up the backbone of support for hurling, Ireland's most traditional sport steeped in a culture of conservative nationalism, they couldn't get a ticket for love, money – or sex – and Vikki's talents on the playing field were not utilised. The fact that Padraig was standing atop the building next door ('More a danger to myself from the 100 pints of porter in me belly than from any notions of topping myself') worried the girls who were in the Kasbah that morning: while never a client of the prostitutes, he was – and still is – a much loved figure among nearly all of them.

Padraig Ó Faoláin was something of a regular renegade from sensible living. A painter of considerable standing, he arrived in the world of the Kasbah after a two-year stay in the Netherlands where his works of modern art were fêted by the Dutch government to the tune of 200 guilders a month – money he spent in the paint-stained company of the canal-side bars of Amsterdam talking with and listening to old men, men in gowns and caps who had talked with and listened to Pablo Picasso.

His trip into bohemian Holland came about as a result of one of the many episodes of mayhem and necessity that marked his life, occurring as it did completely by drunken accident. He had driven a friend out to Dublin Airport to see him off to a new life in Australia – via London. One of the men had miscalculated the departure time by twenty-four hours and, true to form, they returned to one of the terminal's lounges to contemplate their next move. Both men knew each other and themselves well enough to know exactly what that move would be.

'The next thing I can recall with any respectable clarity,' said Padraig, a svelte man with a shock of snow white hair on his face and head who always dresses in black and whose face looks much too troubled and rugged to go with the rest of what God had dealt him, 'was wakening up and seeing my friend puking into a doggy bag. I asked him what was wrong and he said, "I always get sick on planes." I remember shouting out loud for a drink as I tried to convince myself that I was still in the airport lounge.'

The flight saw the two men land safely in London's Heathrow Airport. Padraig's friend made his way on to the continent at the other side of the globe as the bemused artist contemplated the fact that he had just enough money to travel on to Holland, the fare being marginally less than the £16 then needed to return home to Ireland.

He returned to Ireland after a few years, depressed at how badly he felt his art as a painter had suffered while away. Sitting in a hotel in Dublin, he gave me his rationale. 'You know why us – the Irish – are so creative with the words and the paintings and all that? I'll tell you. It's because we do it out of anger and frustration and Ireland is full of that. We do it with our two fingers stuck up to the world; to the begrudgers we see everywhere who think we can't do it. We paint and we write to show them we can do it; we can succeed. We do it out of that anger. We do it to fuck the begrudgers and you can only do that if you are penniless and on the dole in a nation full of begrudgers like Ireland.'

He added, 'And you know what, that anger is justified anger, that's what it is.'

Padraig moved into 59 Mountjoy Square West and was soon a popular figure with the girls next door in the basement bordello. Most mornings he would look down from the high steps and invite the girls who had arrived too early for the morning shift in for tea and sandwiches. Many of them returned his goodwill and gentle companionship by posing for painting sessions in the giant studio he had carved out of the innards of the old building. 'They really were the salt of the earth,' he said. 'Five or six of them would think nothing of climbing onto a bed and having sex with each other for the sake of my painting.'

He was further popularised by his legendary Good Friday parties – one of two days in the Irish calendar when it is legally forbidden to sell alcohol. Padraig had arranged with a Republican gang on the northside of the city to supply him with kegs of draught Guinness and Harp lager for the occasion which he would sell off at £1 per pint. The parties were class-less and creedless affairs – representing a cross section of the society known to the artist, from wealthy 'wannabee' aristo-crats to the hardened inner city types who were his neighbours. The only stipulation for entry – and Padraig insisted on this with uncustomary astringency – was that the men wear formal dress suits and the ladies evening dresses. The rule represented an authentic touch of eccentricity as the hundreds of party goers filed into the large but largely unkempt house on the Square for a night of slightly illegal revelry joined as always by the slightly more illegal ladies of the basement in the adjoining house. 'It's amazing what people will do to have a good time and a drink on a Good Friday. It was class. Real class.'

But the music died for Padraig and the other revellers on Good Friday, 1989, when, at about 5am, he was awoken by a policeman's torch frying his eyes as he slept on the floor where he had crashed out earlier. The officer had made his way in through the front door which was hanging open: he was there out of nothing more serious than professional curiosity. What the two men witnessed when the light was switched on causes Padraig to develop an angry twitch in his neck to this day.

He explained, 'One of the Kasbah women – Vikki – brought her low-life friends to the party and came back when everyone was gone and robbed the place. Then even took my girlfriend's precious operatic tapes. They robbed stuff which was worthless to them yet it was irreplaceable. My girlfriend and I split up shortly afterwards. If I ever meet Vikki again I'll punch her in the fucking face. It gets worse,' he added. 'Before they left they threw all the food against the walls and onto the ceiling. The place was covered in spaghetti Bolognese and fried chicken wings. They destroyed my home.' He added as a kind of footnote to the episode, 'I gave up drink for two years because of that.'

A short time later, Padraig found himself in the unlikely position of pleading for Vikki's life. The Republican beer suppliers got to hear what had happened to his home and took the matter of her punishment into their own hands as a question of honour. 'It took me four meetings with men whose names will go to the grave with me to persuade them not to shoot the bitch dead,' he said. 'They took it all very personal because they felt it was their party as much as mine. I suggested to them that they could break her legs with my eternal blessing or even kneecap her, but Christ almighty, don't kill the woman. They told me the matter was now out of my hands but I must have had some effect because the fucking cow is still around the place as far as I know.'

On the morning of Padraig's encounter with the clouds above Mountjoy Square, Mandy Jameson had pressing problems on her mind. It was 11.30am and, in her own words, 'Beirut was happening outside the front fucking door of the Kasbah': she had borrowed the £15 for her daughter's cake from Vikki who had in turn got the money from the well-known client she had enjoyed looking after earlier that morning. But how was she going to get out? 'The nation's journalists were sitting on top of a brothel with all their cameras and I needed to get out to get my daughter her birthday cake. It was what you might call a dilemma!' Like the good mother she is, Mandy braved the prying throng wrapped in a tweed overcoat she had borrowed from the client. She successfully avoided the cameras and made her way to the cake shop. She already knew that photographers were potentially more dangerous in these situations than reporters who you can always say fuck off and mind your own business to, whereas a photograph can be taken without any consultation and possibly filed for use with a story either that very day (captioned as 'a woman fleeing the building') or some time in the future (captioned as 'a file picture of Ms So And So who was convicted yesterday of vice-related offences', etc.).

For a reason she can't remember (possibly it was to return the coat) Mandy returned to the Kasbah with her daughter's cake as the drama continued to unfold. 'I was doing nicely until this young fella tugged at a photographer and turned pointing at my Jayzuz face and said, "Hey mister, there's one of them whooores from the brottle. Go on, take a picture of her, mister. She's one of dem brottle whooores.' The coat now firmly over her head, the cake under her oxter and travelling at a velocity it was never designed for, Mandy scurried safely back in, not knowing to this day whether the photographer bothered to let off a few shots in her direction or not.

The madness of the morning was completed when a second knock came to the door of the Kasbah while the mayhem out on the street entered its second hour with Padraig still ensconced on the roof, his paintings, his paint and his windows forming their own Picasso-gone-wrong creation on the footpath and the street and the cars below. A bus had crashed by this stage and the road would be closed for four hours. This time the knock on the door was much less impatient that the previous one delivered by the big policeman. It was a client; the day-release patient from St Brendan's Psychiatric Hospital who was a regular at the Kasbah. Charlene could hardly conceal her anger and embarrassment as the client displayed a genuine confusion at not being allowed in.

'Go away,' she hissed. 'Come back later when things have quietened down. Can't you see the cops and the press all over the fucking place?'

He replied, 'Ah, yes, I can see them alright. I see what you mean, alright. But what's that got to do with me coming in now? What's the matter?'

'Look, for fuck's sake, you can't come in now. Fuck off will ya.'

'Okay. But why can't I come in now, Charlene? Can I collect some [blue] videos instead if you won't let me in?'

'*What*? The police are out-fucking-side. Now fuck off.' Charlene's tolerance was worn out.

'I'll give them back. I promise.'

'Look. You. Yeah, you, you little bollocks. *Fuck off.* Now. Go. Now. Get the fuck out of here.'

The client from St Brendan's eventually left and Padraig the artist came down from the building via a non life-threatening route. He appeared in court the following morning and escaped jail despite pleading guilty to seven charges including inciting a riot, resisting arrest, abusive and drunk and disorderly behaviour and causing malicious damage to vehicular traffic. The provisionally set newspaper headlines never married with printer's ink as the evening time deadlines passed with Padraig still ensconced on the roof. Mandy got her cake. The well-known client who'd been inside riding Vikki arrived late for his business meeting but was good humoured and mumbled something about traffic diversions and a delay of some sort up near Mountjoy Square as he took off his tweed coat. The rats in the subterranean sewers had the best Saturday night of their lives.

It was a marginally more eventful day than usual at the Kasbah.

Chapter Sixteen

The Real Poppy Healy

If the fantasies of some men were the realities of the prostitutes of the Kasbah, it was difficult to see how the small, almost frail-looking woman with the mousey-blonde hair and the soft accent honed in the rural spa lands of Berrings, County Cork, was going to fit in, both with clients and with some of the hard-bitten, violent-tongued women of Ireland's most infamous bordello.

Yet within weeks of her arrival towards the end of July 1988, Margaret 'Poppy' Healy had proven herself a formidable woman, a survivor among her kind, grudgingly admired as someone who played to her strengths, but equally despised by her contemporaries as being wantonly vindictive and petty minded. Little could anyone have realised that Poppy Healy – through playing to those strengths and relieving one client alone of over £12,000 in an eight-month period – would be instrumental in dismantling the Kasbah and with it over a decade of highly original vice in Ireland when she testified against her former employer and good friend, Marion Murphy, in front of a judge and jury in the Central Criminal Court in February 1993.

Like most of her contemporaries, Margaret Healy got into the vice game in response to financial pressures. She had worked in a hotel in Cork before coming to Dublin in late 1986 to begin her new career as a prostitute. While employed as a barmaid she received generous tips from a visiting eminent clergyman who stayed at the hotel and would look for Ms Healy's company for his late night drinks. Neither she nor anyone else in the nation could have foreseen the spectacular fall from grace of the much loved and ebullient churchman over the Annie Murphy love-child scandal as Poppy and the Bishop spent the small hours drinking and giggling in obvious delight with each other's company.

The Bishop of Galway, The Most Reverend Dr Eamonn Casey, would insist that Maggie, as he was fond of calling her, keep the change from each new £5 note he proffered for his alcoholic spirit. While forthcoming with his bank-roll and his compliments for his caterer, the relationship between the then thirty-six-year-old Maggie Healy and her conversation-loving clerical companion never extended beyond the harmless enclosures of the hotel lounge and residents' bar.

Margaret Healy spent her first two years in Dublin working in two of the thirty-eight brothels fronting as massage parlours which were operating in the city at that time. She was introduced to Linda Lavelle and the Kasbah on the word of a girl who used the trade name Julie and who was employed from time to time by Linda. In her statement of evidence to the police investigating the Kasbah during 1991 she said she spent the first two weeks of her employment in the Kasbah opening the main door in the mornings, cleaning and lighting the fire, sorting out linen, towels, etc. She worked under the name 'Carol', given to her, she claimed to the police, by Marion Murphy. (She was given the nickname 'Poppy' after a blazing row with the Kasbah's unofficial cook, gay Gladys, who accused her of spreading rumours about one of his many platonic girlfriends. 'Poppy' was a reference to the Irish radio show, *Aunty Poppy Story Time* and was a bitchy and somewhat undeserved reference to Ms Healy's penchant for telling tales).

'Initially,' Poppy would later tell police, 'I didn't get involved with the clients.' She said she started taking men for sex because Marion Murphy wasn't paying her some pre-arranged chore-money. Whether or not the claim was true, it did serve to point up the deep rift which had developed between herself and Marion, her one-time boss and confidante. (Once, to the astonishment of other prostitutes in the Kasbah, Poppy 'looked after' three clients in a row who were only willing to pay the minimum £15 entrance fee in return for topless relief, a euphemism for masturbation. Such minimum payments went directly to the madam who would hand back £3 on each booking to the girls. Margaret Healy did the work willingly. 'Isn't it money?' she told them in her Corkonian lilt. 'Isn't money there – £45 book money there for Marion?')

And while some of the prostitutes might be slow to admit it today, Poppy Healy had earned at least the professional respect of the prostitutes who worked the Kasbah. Linda Lavelle herself had opined, 'The best girl is the one to be fit to put on the act – that is what is meant by being good at what you're at in this line of work.' And of Margaret Healy she once said, 'She was a plain looking woman and she knew what category she fitted into and what she would have to do [to make money] and she did it. She knew what she had to do to be popular with a certain type of client because there was no way she was going to be popular with them all. Poppy gave what I'd call total impression: she acted in the rooms as if she was enjoying it – as though she wasn't being paid – in that respect she was the best type of girl.'

But whatever bank of goodwill Poppy Healy had generated by her occasional and apparent selfless acts for her Madam, it all evaporated quickly. For Poppy was perceived to have had a streak of spiteful malice which could only be borne out of a woman who was either emotionally hurt or emotionally unstable, or both. It wasn't long before she had become the target for criticism and some isolation among the other girls. Ironically, she was also looked upon as a lesser-type; a lower form of prostitute, insofar as she became involved in practices with clients that even the 'total whores' – as Vikki was fond of referring to herself and some of her pals – often baulked at. It was Margaret Healy who often fed Smelly Bottoms the actor his own faeces with matchsticks from a plate in a back room at the Kasbah. It was Margaret Healy and Mandy Jameson who took on most of the clients who dealt in that most awful world of sexual gratification through the use of human excrement.

While privately denigrated for dealing with these clients, the criticisms of her by the others girls were, I felt throughout my research, both unnecessarily cruel and hypocritical: Poppy had long since shown that she was no match for Vikki, Pia, Mandy, Charlene, Susan, Hayley, Linda and others when it came to so-called straight customers. She was playing to her strengths, that's all, and that was the only standard the girls themselves measured each other by. Said Pia, 'I could go into a room with a client planning to spend £20 and walk out forty minutes later with a £100 in my bra. If the same man were to come back next week with the same money to spend and Poppy did him she'd be lucky to get out of there with a stiff or a chicken. [Trade terms for a wank or masturbation, £5; and the minimum book price for a massage, £15.] 'Poppy knew that: she knew she'd have to go after the dirty bastards, the scumbags with the shite and the dirty fingers if she was going to make a living at this game because none of the other punters really wanted her. And it wasn't down to her plain looks: it was down to the fact that she whined so much and often tried to contact clients when they were outside the Kasbah in the real world. No one will stand for that if they've an ounce of cop on.'

Poppy's many differences with her fellow travellers in the Kasbah were typified by an incident there on a Saturday morning sometime towards the end of 1989 while working a shift with Pia who explained, 'We were particularly busy. Me and Poppy were on duty and, as usual, Poppy wasn't getting many of the clients. I was so busy that I was hopping from room to room looking after clients with just a towel around my arse – I was so busy that I didn't have time to get dressed after each session. I was minting it! Poppy was sitting in the front room brooding away. She let another client in and told him to go to the back room. She told me he was looking for me. I felt sorry for her and I told the client that I was up to my eyes and would he mind taking Carol [Poppy] instead and he said okay. But she was already fuming and wouldn't have anything to do with it.'

Pia continued, 'She told me, "How the Hell am I supposed to get any of the clients when you're traipsing around the place dropping the towel in front of the clients and asking them if you could look after them?"

'I told her not to be stupid. I told her to go down to the end room and just tell the client I'm busy and do him yourself. I was really freaking out with her at this stage but I tried not to show it. She refused and I blew me top. "Look," I told her, "he's your fucking client. You booked him in. He's your responsibility. Now do the cunt and stop fucking around for Jesus' sake."'

The next thing Pia remembers was getting up off the floor, her head spinning as she punched the digits of Linda Lavelle's home telephone. 'You know what the fucking bitch is after doing, Linda. She's after slapping me across the face. There's going to be trouble down here, Linda.' Pia's temper, while not easily stoked, was dynamite. The would-be client in the bottom room sat there, his ardour waning by the minute as the two women kept at it.

'I'm not doing him, Poppy. I'm not doing the cunt.'

'Well you should let him out then, girl. You're the one dropping the towel. You know that's shameless.' (Poppy's lapses into moral sharp shooting were legendary.)

'No, Poppy, he's your client. You took the [book] money from him.'

Neither woman was aware that by this stage a third party had joined them and was trying to get a word in edge ways. It was the client. 'Look-et,' he said in his mild Dublin accent. 'I'll leave and that'll solve the problem, roight?' The punter headed out the door and up the basement steps, forgetting to ask for his book money back. That he had had two hookers fighting over him in a brothel would have been little consolation.

The treatment of the bemused client was, of course, just part of a sideshow, a handle on which to hang the pent-up frustrations felt by Pia and so many of the Kasbah girls towards Margaret 'Poppy' Healy. But however much Pia disliked Poppy, their many altercations never scaled the Machiavellian heights Vikki was capable of operating on, as the faltering Cork woman found out when the two of them were working a shift together on another occasion and a knock came to the door.

'I looked out the peep-hole,' recalled Vikki, 'and I said to Poppy that we shouldn't let this little gurrier in. I told her he looked like a burglar. She said don't be silly, it was a client and he didn't look like a burglar to her. Anyways, I opened the door and let him in. He turned out to be a nice kind of chap. Quiet. When he took a look at me and Poppy he decided he wanted to screw me. Fair enough. So I takes him to one of the rooms and we were chatting away when I noticed him take out two sawn-off ends of 7-UP cans and put them on top of the television as cool as you like and I asked him what they were for. He said, "Look, I'll do my job and you do yours." Then he told me he was a housebreaker. Fuck . . . I was right all along, but I said to myself, "That's grand, he'll probably have lots of readies if he's after coming from a job. I'll get a few quid out of this geezer."'

Vikki continued as she lit up another cigarette using the

ashes of the previous one to light it, 'He started to strip off his underwear and I started to fucking shake, I mean fucking tremble. He was covered in abscesses. Some had plasters on them, some were still weeping and some were lanced. He was the most fucked-up looking strung-out junkie I've ever seen. I was really afraid of this guy because his type fly off the handle for no reason at all. I was afraid to refuse him sex yet there was no way I was going to go down on top of a strung-out junkie like him, condom or no fucking condom.'

By this time Vikki's mind was racing as the client now known in vice lore as The Scabby Burglar unwittingly provided her with the way out she was desperately looking for when he asked, 'Do you do full sex?'

'Oh, Jesus, sorry, luv,' came the mightily relieved reply. (Vikki recalled the incident with, what was for her, unusual clarity.) 'When he asked about full sex as if he expected I mightn't be into it I thought to myself, "Halle-e-fucking-luja, I can escape in one piece."'

The conversation continued.

'You want full sex? Jesus, luv, I'm really so sorry. I don't do full sex, It's just a personal thing I do have about full sex. Couldn't live with meself, luv. You know how it is with the husband and kids. I thought you were only looking for a wank or something. But don't worry, luv, there's a girl just outside who'll look after you. I'll send her in right away.'

Vikki left the room hot foot and found Poppy where she always was, at the roaring fire in the big front room. 'Poppy, he wants you to do him. He doesn't want me at all.' Inscrutable, Ms Healy responded to the request and headed in. As soon as Vikki heard the door close she bolted out and up onto the street to look for help and in so doing headed straight into yet another near calamitous drama. She said, 'Five or six fellas in cars started honking their horns and bursting their guts laughing at me. I hadn't realised it at the time but I was still in working clothes, red shoes, a tiny red leather mini-skirt and a

white see-through blouse [no bra]. I'm not sure if I was wearing any knickers at the time but if I was they would have been
micro.' The highly entertained motorists could have told her
as she ran up the high steps to the main door of Number
60B, exposing the rear end of her anatomy to the world as she
bashed on the door looking for the landlord or any of the
tenants to come in and give Poppy a digout with this 'mad
bastard' inside. Across the street Linda Lavelle was in a similar
state of amusement as Vikki, not for the first time, was giving
a free and unwitting preview of what life could be like in the
Kasbah for those who dared venture in. She said, 'I crossed
over as quick as I could and headed straight for the Kasbah. I
was met by Poppy racing towards the door in panic and The
Scabby Burglar behind her zipping up his trousers. "Linda,
Linda,"' she said, "I've got AIDS, I've got AIDS. He raped me.
I've been raped."'

For months afterwards, Margaret Healy talked about the
night she was raped by a burglar. I wondered whether it was
the guilty ghosts of her Catholic conscience being dealt with
by extreme denial of what she had become – a prostitute – or
whether she actually was violated physically and otherwise by
the client. Only she can answer. Or, perhaps, she can't answer.
One way or the other, she received little sympathy from her
colleagues. 'Poppy's Poppy. She was always carrying on with
some fucking sob story or another. She was always acting the
martyr,' said one of them.

As fate would have it, Poppy and Vikki were to encounter
another burglar during a shift together at the Kasbah – only
this one was on active service. Vikki tells the story. 'It was a
strange sort of situation. I opened the door and this mad looking geezer held a bottle up to my face and demanded money.
Poppy came out and started screaming to high fuck. The whole
of Mountjoy Square could have heard her. The burglar got a bit
jumpy with all the noise and looked like he was preparing to do
a runner out of the place. Poppy continued screaming but the

fucker couldn't get out again because I had locked him in. You always lock the door before and after clients. Here was this big fucker charging around the place with a broken bottle in his hand trying to get out, roaring to get out, and Poppy still screaming her lungs out. I realised that it was only a matter of time before it dawned on him that Poppy's screaming wasn't exactly causing the fucking Light Brigade to come charging in to save us: sooner or later he'd realise that it was just him, me and Poppy and that he could do what he liked to us.' The situation was defused when Vikki managed to unlock the large steel front door and throw it open. Like a trapped rat, the panic-stricken burglar spotted the grudging shaft of daylight and made a run for it. He had managed to lift £400 in cash, none of it Vikki's. That night in the pub Poppy remained silent as if in shock. All Vikki seemed genuinely hurt by was the loss of a packet containing three Major cigarettes.

'The cunt stole me fags. That bastardin' cunt stole me last cigarettes.'

In July 1990 Poppy had taken what she deemed was enough abuse from Vikki and she called the police after the pair had become involved in a dust-up in a hotel not far from the Kasbah. The problem this time, however, was that the pair of them were in the Canary Islands off the west coast of Africa, courtesy of a drink-troubled and very wealthy client of Vikki's who had convinced himself that he was in love with her. And this time the police had guns and seemed quite prepared to use them if necessary. (The Kasbah in question was the well-known shopping centre in Gran Canaria from which Linda Lavelle had taken the name for what became Ireland's best known whore house.)

Said Vikki, 'The only reason Poppy was invited was because my client Paul [not his real name] was travelling with friends from his business. He was a country lad and wanted to make out that Poppy was his cousin who he was treating. I was

supposed to be Poppy's friend from Dublin whom she had
agreed to take along to keep her company. But he boasted to
his mates that I was really nuts about him and that I wanted
him to leave the wife and shack up with me. He used to tell
them that he would have nothing to do with me; that I was a
common little slut from Dublin.'

Paul, whose wife is well known and very wealthy in her
own right, was a relatively big spender. Not only did he foot
the flight and hotel bills for the two Kasbah prostitutes, he also
gave Vikki £200 sterling in Spain and a further cheque for
£350 in Irish punts as they got off the plane in Dublin six days
later. 'It was a pretty good trip except for Margaret Healy,' said
Vikki. 'I only screwed Paul twice because we were a few miles
away from where he and his mates were staying and we had to
get the midnight bus back. Midnight I ask you: two whores in
bed by 12am on their Spanish holiday, I ask you! Once or
twice I got Poppy to come into the clubs with me as soon as
we got back, just for one drink. I told her that she needn't
stay – just one drink to help me mingle with the crowd and
then she could fuck off to bed. One night Paul came over to
the club with the boys and joined us. The crack was great: a
couple of German guys were out of their minds pissed. They
started pulling down their trousers and flashing their arses
and I was busy minding me own business taking holiday snaps
of them. Suddenly Poppy started to complain about me to
Paul but he said to her to leave me alone; that I was just having a bit of harmless fun. Then – typical Poppy – she starts
giving out to me there and then, telling me I should have
more respect for Paul and for myself. After all, says she, he was
the one paying for my holiday.

'After the club closed me and Poppy were making our way
up the stairs of the hotel on our own when she started giving
out a-fucking-gain. I lost me reason. I went for the jugular.
I smashed her about the place right and good. I thought
that was the end of it until a bit later when I got a knock on

the bedroom door and here were these two uniformed Spanish policemen with guns trying to tell me they were investigating a complaint of assault regarding me and another woman.'

The incident was resolved without a single shot being fired. The flight home was without incident: the cheque for £350 was given by Paul to Vikki discreetly in the airport terminal at Dublin. He promised he'd phone soon.

A few weeks later he called Vikki at the (Irish) Kasbah and told her that he had left the wife and kids and would she meet him for a drink to discuss things. Never slow to spot the chance of some handy readies – and perennially in dire need of same – Vikki agreed, even though she knew she was breaking one of the unwritten rules among the prostitutes: getting involved between a client and his wife. Vikki had no idea she was being watched as she sat in his car outside the pub powdering her cheeks and applying her 'total whore' red lipstick while he went inside and ordered two large brandies. She waggled over to the high stools in the crowded bar where she knew Paul would be: he always positioned himself within reaching distance of the alcohol dispensers.

'How's it going, kid?' (Vikki remembers Paul looking 'very down, serious and depressed'.)

'Grand, Paul. What's going on? Something wrong?'

'I've left Mary [not her real name] and the kids, Vikki . . . [he actually called her by her real Christian name] and . . .'

Vikki had barely got the brandy glass to her blazing-red lips when a tall, good-looking woman in her mid forties joined them. Paul hid whatever sense of surprise he may have experienced very well.

'Vikki, this is my wife.'

The Dublin prostitute turned around slowly, not knowing what to expect and realising right away that she had been followed, or, worse, Paul had set the whole thing up. 'Pleased to meet you.'

The woman looked at Vikki stony faced, her back to her husband. She pointed to a face in the crowded bar, addressing both of them but keeping her eyes locked on Vikki's before completing her husband's family introduction.

'. . . and that there, that girl there is our daughter. Paul's daughter.' Vikki remembers that the woman was by now trembling with rage.

'There are three other children at home. I am Paul's wife. Paul is my husband. Do you understand?'

The Dublin prostitute had been around too many corners in her life to know that honesty can be a fairweather friend when the atmosphere is laced with lies and deceit and infidelity. Like the American warlords in Vietnam, the time had come to declare victory and retreat.

'I'm a friend of Paul's, that's all,' she lied unconvincingly. 'Why are you telling me all of this?'

Paul turned to his wife, 'Look, I've just bought this girl a drink, for Heaven's sake. Can we not all sit down here in a civilised way and just talk about . . .'

Perhaps, I thought, his wife had heard him play that tune one time too many. Or perhaps seeing the evidence, the flesh and bones, of something always denied by him and that she had denied to herself had made that expression of innocence impossible to accept now. Vikki recalls what happened next with more of her unaccustomed clarity 'The poor woman fucking exploded. You can sing that, baby . . . she ex-fucking-ploded in the middle of the pub. I felt sorry for Paul. A bit, anyway.' Her sympathy did not manifest itself in support, however. She reckoned quite rightly that getting a few quid from Paul right then in front of his missus would be both fruitless and indelicate.

'I guess I'll be off,' she said as she eased herself off the bar stool.

'No!' said Paul, holding her by the wrist. 'You're not going anywhere. I want you to listen to this.'

At this stage her high-spending high flying client's tactic had moved from injured innocence to vicious counter attack. It was classic crisis management and, of course, it blew what was left of his cover.

Paul and his wife have subsequently legally separated. His personal disintegration has since become complete with chronic addiction to alcohol and the deluded state of mind that goes with it. Because of a perverse kind of honour, he no longer has anything to do with Vikki. He ditched her when he found out that she had had a steady boyfriend for years: the traitor betrayed, a bit like Lauden the diplomat with Linda Lavelle.

He could, however, be grateful to one woman. If it hadn't been for Margaret Healy's purportedly 'difficult decision' to tell him all about two-timing Vikki, he might never have found out the truth.

A real friend was Poppy, he reasoned.

The episode of Vikki, Poppy, and Mr and Mrs Paul more poignantly than others throws up issues that I have been studiously attempting avoid in the writing of this book: issues of victims, real and imagined; of the validity or otherwise of the patriarchy standpoint; of abuse and of morality. My own views on this were much more clear-cut before I started out on this book. I saw the prostitutes as the victims and men – both the clients and male society in general – as the perpetrators, the victimisers. Those views are now displaced by no views; by my confusion. Searching for victims and deciding where the blame resides in the world of hired sex is for me both a shallow and fraudulent task because it implies a difference: some women are prostitutes and some are not; some men are their clients and some are not.

It was a way of thinking I used which I wasn't even aware of and which ensured that, as a non-prostitute and non-client, I had no need to be challenged, threatened or otherwise engaged by prostitution. But what if there was no *difference* between me and the prostitutes or me and the clients? What if my life had taken a left instead of a right turn somewhere down the way which led me to the door of a bordello? Am I so fundamentally different that I can say that that would never happen to me? Much more difficult and valid is the proposition that this whole issue is about casualties, victims of the human condition and of the circumstances life throws up. Poppy Healy, Vikki O'Toole, Mr Paul, his wife, their children, are all casualties of circumstance and with that we can all identify to a lesser or greater extent because we are all victims of some sort or another.

The difficulty I have with this, with viewing people, their humanity and their circumstance in this way, is that there are no simple explanations and no solutions: there is no no-man's-land between them and me. There is no way I can distance myself anymore. And there is no way I should.

Such thoughts, however, were unlikely to have been troubling Vikki as she pondered the prospect that Paul and his ready money had dried up since he had learnt the truth about 'the other man'. Whatever motives Poppy Healy had for telling Paul, they count for nothing in the vice business: motive is not important, money is. And Margaret Healy had once again shown her apparent bloody-minded knack for screwing things up for herself and others.

Vikki and Mandy (and, of course, Linda Lavelle) were not the only women in the Kasbah to fall victims to Poppy Healy's strange and troubled behaviour. Mandy had been doing very nicely thank you out of a client from rural Ireland who had business interests in Dublin and who the girls called The Candy Man. He was a Discipline client, 'A dirty man who didn't wash himself that often and who was definitely getting worse with his perversions as the years passed on,' according to his hired woman. But The Candy Man paid well and when Mandy ran into difficulties raising money for a deposit on her first house, he was not found wanting. 'He put £1,000 in my bank account, that's the way things worked between us. There'd be weeks where he wouldn't pay but I was always sure of getting my money – good money. And anytime I asked for a dig-out with a bill or whatever he'd come across with the cash. You've got to look after a man like that,' said Mandy.

As with the disintegrating figure of Paul and his prostitute Vikki, The Candy Man was not aware that there was a permanent man in Mandy's life, not, anyway, until Margaret Healy told him, and further explained that the house was for Mandy, her husband and their children (which was not strictly accurate because fate had long since parted her from her legal spouse). 'I'm still very bitter about that,' Mandy says. 'There was no call for her ruining things between me and a good client, a client who I could get £400 or £500 off of regularly.' As if to rub salt into the wounds, The Candy Man contacted Margaret Healy shortly after the Garda raid which led to her conviction on 13 May 1992 for running a brothel at 60B Mountjoy Square West offering her a new life out of the city. He set her up with an apartment and a job in one of his several small business ventures in a large provincial town. Eventually, Margaret Healy ended up in Britain where she worked in a clerical position with a privately-owned energy company.

Poppy Healy's disputatiousness always carried with it that curious moral tone: with Mandy, she felt that The Candy Man wasn't getting a fair deal; that he was somehow being duped by a dishonest and immoral woman who was two-timing him. On another occasion she chided Mandy for taking money from Smelly Bottoms the actor and failing to turn up for a late night session of scatological deviance in return for the fee. (She even once advised Smelly Bottoms to stop coming to the Kasbah – to girls like herself and Mandy – and to seek psychiatric help instead to get himself straightened out, whatever that meant. 'The fucking cheek of her,' Mandy said later.

'Imagine telling a good customer to go elsewhere. Sure hadn't *we* got what Smelly was looking for? Didn't *we* look after him? The fucking cheek of her.')

Poppy's vexed and freewheeling righteousness took on new heights when she and four other prostitutes from the Kasbah travelled south to the wedding of the nurse, Lorraine, the girl who had spent six months working at the brothel in the late 1980s (see p.139). Lorraine and Linda Lavelle had become close friends – a relationship not lost on Poppy. During the car journey to the wedding in a County Cork town she lost no opportunity in assuring Lorraine that she had made a big mistake in inviting the other girls, Mandy, Vikki and Pia.

'They're whores and they'll let you down. They'll ruin your big day for sure,' she counselled. 'Everyone in [the county] is going to know that Lorraine worked as a whore.'

Linda, Mandy, Poppy and Pia booked three rooms in the hotel where the reception was due to be held. Poppy spent the entire night, according to the girls, on point duty at the door. The following morning over breakfast she castigated Mandy and Vikki for having men in the room. 'I told Lorraine that ye pair would ruin it. Ye can't keep away from men and their money.'

Poppy was right about the men being in the room but they could hardly be described as clients: they were Mandy's two brothers. They lived close by and when they learnt that she'd be in town had gone over to the hotel and spent the bleary hours imploring their sister for the umpteenth time to turn from her sinful ways which could bring untold dishonour to the entire family, including her venerated aunty nuns. (Although she was genuinely pleased to see them, Mandy was drunk and kept telling both of them to fuck off without really meaning it. Vikki, being a city girl and having no such experience of brotherly concern – hopeless or not – just soaked in this strange sibling experience as she sweetened up the room with the fragrances of her beloved 'wacky baccy'.)

The weekend turned out to be a gas. Said Linda, 'Everyone was pissed for the entire three days. It was a grand old country wedding and the crack was mighty. Lorraine's father knew that she had worked as a prostitute in the Kasbah and didn't seem to mind a bit. He knew we were all Kasbah women and had a field day trying to fix us up for the night with some of the old, backward country folk during the dancing. He was a real leg puller. He introduced Vikki as one of Lorraine's best friends and told everyone that the three of us were single and looking for men! He fixed Pia up with a big old farmer who lost the run of himself with manners and good behaviour. Jesus, we were swamped by them. If they only fucking knew the type of women they were dancing with! If they only knew that all the bridal gear had been made in a fucking brothel in Dublin by an old grannie prostitute!'

Margaret Healy spent the three days at the bar, ignored by everyone and alone. She was being punished by her fellow prostitutes and she seemed if not comfortable in that role then certainly familiar with it. It was difficult to believe that this was the same woman who took a bunch of flowers from a fellow prostitute – a gift from a client called Dirty Don – only minutes after climbing naked from underneath the dead John Bones and placed them on the corpse as she prayed for his spiritual deliverance; vowing to give up this awful business of prostitution; vowing never to go into that room again and then, later that same night, having sex with a client in that room as if nothing had happened. She was and still is a woman much easier to ridicule than to understand. 'Poppy gloated on sympathy. She gloated on having to go for an AIDS test,' said Pia. 'I think she actually enjoyed being short-changed by a client because then she had something to moan about. She needed to have something to complain about and if she didn't then she'd become spiteful and she'd do the dirty on any of us, it really didn't matter which one of us. She was on some kind of ego-sympathy trip.'

Linda Lavelle is more astringent. 'Margaret Healy wanted to own the Kasbah. I knew I should have thrown her out years ago. She had become too powerful. She had got enough inside knowledge to destroy me and the Kasbah. She was glad to leave when she had got rid of the Kasbah because if she could not have it then she did not want me to have it. In that sense I played a part in my own downfall in that I didn't do something about getting rid of her shortly after she arrived when she started showing signs of the person she turned out to be.'

From the view in the press box in the Circuit Criminal Court on Wednesday, 5 February 1993, the frail-looking woman with the lank, grey hair and the glasses looked more like a nun let out for the first time in twenty years than a convicted forty-two-year-old prostitute. How could such a manifestly lethargic person evoke such a wealth of resentment and ill will from her former colleagues? Both senior counsel Kevin Haugh, appearing for Marion Murphy, and the State's barrister Shane Murray, were clearly exasperated by her performance in the witness box. Time and time again she appeared not to want to answer the simplest questions.

'Were you paid for having sex? Are you a prostitute? Was Marion Murphy aware of what was going on in the Kasbah? How many women worked at the Kasbah?'

Her answers were monosyllabic and constipated. Judge Gerard Buchanan showed sympathetic patience. Ms Healy was obviously extremely uncomfortable at being there: whether she was a reluctant witness against her former pal was only for her to know.

One inescapable truth, however, was that she was there, however reluctantly, and with each one of her affirmations she drove another nail into the coffin of the Kasbah and the women who worked there. Marion Murphy, the woman accused of brothel-keeping at the Kasbah, sat just ten feet from where Margaret 'Poppy' Healy gave her evidence, alone and directly opposite the jury at the foot of a courtroom wall that seemed to stretch to the sky and I couldn't help thinking that if Poppy Healy felt isolated and frightened and naked in the light just then, it was nothing compared to what Marion Murphy was going through.

Maybe, just maybe, this was the real Margaret Healy.

Chapter Seventeen

Dangerous Liaisons

The price of victory is not cheap
And with you I long to sleep
Give me peace and give me rest
Give me comfort at your breast

The sun was splitting the trees on the afternoon of 28 May 1990 as the entire nation was caught up in the fever-grip of the Irish soccer squad's elevation to the final rounds of the World Cup which were to be played out in Italy in less than two weeks' time. Not since Pope John Paul II's visit to Ireland in 1979 had the population experienced such a groundswell of pride and positive self-image. That the team had been moulded together by an Englishman after successive Irish managers had demonstrably failed to take Ireland barely beyond international soccer's Third Division didn't matter a damn: Jack Charlton was a national hero. Arguably, he had done more for national self-esteem than any of the great leaders of modern Irish history.

Down at the Islamic Centre on the South Circular Road, passers-by – many of them wearing the national white, green and gold World Cup bunting and accessories – paid little attention to one young man as he stepped out of the taxi cab and took off his shoes before entering the Islamic mosque. They could not have known of the racist anger welling inside him, and neither could his foreign hosts as they showed him around the sacred temple of prayer. John Keegan had no interest in Islam, just a curiosity and concern that they seemed to be recruiting a lot of white women these days.

The conversation in the mosque was curious and courteous and brief. He had seen all he wanted to see. It was only when he got back into the taxi waiting to return him to the city centre that his true racist colours were hoisted full mast. The young fare had no time for foreigners including these Islamic sorts, no time at all: they had no right coming into Ireland and taking our women, he opined to the rear view head and shoulders of the taxi driver. It was about time someone took a stand and expressed how everyone else really felt about the matter, he said.

Like cabbies the world over, the driver had developed a mental sponge for such talk and responded in tones fitting to someone who was partially paying his wages.

'Game ball to you, son. You're dead fucking right. If there were more people standin' up to them A-rabs and I-raneeans we'd be better off. We're only a nation of hypocrites for not speaking up for ourselves. Sure how could that crowd in Iran be right after being poisoned by that Ayatolla Khomeini fella. Game ball. Fair dues to ya.'

If the same cabbie had had a disciple of Islam in the back of his large Toyota saloon earlier that morning he would surely have been welcoming him to Ireland such was his ability to get on with clientele of every hue.

'We're the salt of the earth once you get to know us. Love our pint of Arthur Guinness and like our women. We've nothing against coloureds and, er, blacks. Game ball, me oul flower. Game ball, that's us.'

The young man in the back of the cab cruising down Camden Street heading into the city centre was flush with cash. He had taken up a severance offer from An Post, the Irish Post Office, where he had worked for years in a clerical position.

For the time being at least, he could spend, spend, spend his way out of his own self loathing.

'Where are you headed, son?'

'Oh, anywhere. Back into town I suppose.'

'I know a place where you can get a girl, a nice Irish girl. Don't be worrying about them A-rab and Moslem fellas. There'll be none of them around to bother you in this place.'

A few minutes later the two men headed down the iron steps of the Kasbah, the taxi driver first. Linda Lavelle opened the door as the cabbie cupped his hand around his lips, away from his fare. 'I have a customer for you,' he whispered. 'Here. How much is in it for me?' The two knew each other and had carried on similar conversations before. A small group of taxi men in the city regularly brought potential clients to the Kasbah in return for commission. 'Leave him here with us and call back later,' said Linda. That's all he needed to hear. The customer would, of course, pay the taxi man twice because whatever prostitute looked after him would charge him a tenner or so over the odds to cover the commission. The young man moved closer to the intimacy of words going on between the two. 'I think he wants a massage', said the driver. 'I think a massage and maybe a bit more,' he added with a wink.

The young man opened his mouth for the first time. 'Yeah,' he said casually but with confidence, 'it's actually a ride I'm looking for.'

The prostitutes who were listening in from behind the bottle-green curtain could spot a 'greener' from 10,000 feet and this one bore all the hallmarks of someone on his first visit to a brothel. The young would-be customer did, in fact, know of the Kasbah's existence having spotted an advertisement for the place in *Executive* magazine back in 1982 during his search for sexual encounters. In his naivety, he was unable to decipher the obvious codes like 'thorough massage', 'warm friendly atmosphere', 'all tastes catered for', and 'attractive and friendly female staff to make you feel really relaxed'. He took no comfort from the prospect (as he perceived it) of a straightforward massage, even if it was from a 'friendly female'.

Poppy Healy was on duty that day and it was her turn to take a client who wasn't specifying preferences. 'Hi, I'm Carol,' she said in her sometimes squeaky Cork accent as she stood in front of him wearing only a one-piece black swimsuit. 'Can I look after you?' John Keegan followed the smallish woman behind the bottle-green curtain and down the hall. He was immediately taken with her ampleness and, much more importantly, her blonde hair. He guessed she was about forty and his eyes were rolling at the thought of descending somewhere warm, deep down between those magnificent child-bearing hips. John Keegan was a virgin as he walked through the doors of the Kasbah. He was also a deeply mentally disturbed man, although never physically dangerous. He was something of an emotional and sexual castaway who thought that he had just fallen in love.

Keegan remembers that first coupling vividly. 'I do remember Margaret . . . I said, "How much?" and she said forty pounds. She started going on about whether she'd do it in Swedish or French which was all lost on me because I didn't know what she was talking about because all I wanted was sex, straight sex as far as I can get it. Margaret warmed me up a little bit first. "Why don't you take off your clothes," she said. Margaret started working on me. Then she climbed on top of me and all the time she was on top of me she was saying, "Do you like that?" I was in heaven.

'It was all over in about five minutes.'

From that very first encounter, Keegan felt that he had been shortchanged by Margaret Healy, not realising that he was paying the taxi man's commission through her. ('But what I didn't know was that she was charging £10 above the going rate. Because the going rate was only £30.')

A short time later the cabbie dropped John Keegan outside his home in Clontarf and had the brass to ask his fare for an extra £5. 'Did I think it was worth it, he asked me. I didn't mind giving him another few quid because I was happy and I was singing and there was no shortage of money in those days.'

Later John Keegan added, 'My relationship with Margaret developed simply because we did so much business together. I mean, I was with her over 200 times and she was my stable sex partner if you like. Most of the encounters in the Kasbah were with Margaret Healy, although there were a couple with Linda who took me to the sauna once and said to me, "Did you ever sweat with a woman? Well, you will today." She was fooling around with me in the sauna and eventually it got too hot so she took me out and we went onto the bed. We were trying to have sex there but the bed had a dreadful squeak so she put a towel around her bottom and she lay on the floor and we had sex on the floor. That's the most memorable sex session I think I ever had with her. I had sex with Linda about twelve times, but, em, the bulk of my sexual activity was with Margaret.'

Linda Lavelle remembers thinking after only a few weeks after Keegan's anchorage with Poppy, 'I don't know what he wanted or felt he should get. I don't know where Margaret Healy thought it was going or where it would get her. I was fucking worried about this, this thing between them. They were nutty and this thing they had was nutty and I didn't like it.'

If John Keegan was looking for love then he would have guessed quickly that he had come to the right place. The fact that he had just left his job with the Post Office and was given £12,000 in settlement ensured that he'd get all the love Poppy Healy – and once or twice some other girls at the Kasbah – could give him. For the first time in his troubled life, he had felt emotionally 'owned' by someone – by Poppy Healy. He was glad that he had given up his job because the boredom of it was driving him around the bend. Now he had money and freedom and the two awful stints he had spent in psychiatric care in Dublin in 1988 and the following year were behind him. His mother had long since given up trying to understand her John, although she loved him dearly. She put up with his idiosyncrasies like turning the bedroom of the small terraced house in the north city suburb of Clontarf into a gallery of hand painted murals of clothed and semi-clothed women; always blonde, just like Margaret 'Poppy' Healy. And his mother had no idea of the blame and the anger he harboured for her deep within himself because of what he saw as his dismal failure in establishing himself with members of the opposite sex.

Until the time he had sex with Margaret Healy in one of the tiny back rooms at the brothel in Mountjoy Square, the nearest John Keegan had got to a woman was in the inner city's North Star Hotel where he had managed to steal a kiss on the cheek from a young barmaid who had just invited him to her twenty-first party. (The party itself was a disaster. Keegan's sister and her friend had lined him up with a blind date whom he studiously ignored for the whole night as he ogled the birthday girl, fantasising where a journey starting with a perfectly innocent kiss might end. At the end of the night he was left in that most familiar position: no blind date, no barmaid dream girl, just familiar isolation.)

Eight months after his somewhat fateful first taxi ride to the Kasbah, John Keegan – by then he gloried in the name the girls had given to him of Little John – lived in the charabanc of freedom; freedom from himself. He had fallen head over heels in infatuation, and perhaps in love, for a woman called Margaret 'Poppy' Healy. He would call at the Kasbah three or four times a week, often stopping there all day waiting to take Poppy off on a deluded dalliance as soon as her shift finished. They would go drinking in local hotels, including the Waldorf on the quays of the Liffey. He had developed a real liking for large bottles of Guinness while Poppy was a long-time convert to Power's Irish whiskey and ginger ale.

Sometimes he would spend nights in her home in Rathfarnham, a comfortable middle-class suburb about five miles south of the river. They would drink coffee and vodka and whiskey together in the kitchen downstairs. He would love it when she called him 'honey' before they both headed off to the Kasbah in her shiny new black Renault 19 car, bought, partially at least, on the strength of her trade with her front seat passenger.

He remembered one night in November 1990 being in Poppy's place when there were two women on his mind, one of whom was destined to become one of the great figureheads of Irish life and who was already something of a champion for women's rights as she sought election to the country's highest office. 'Poppy brought me out to the house and she cooked me a big steak,' he said. 'On the table was a big farmer's dinner and then she said would I like a drink and I said no, I didn't really want to go out. The whole idea was to have sex in the house with her. As I had said to Linda at the time, I would like to sleep with Margaret as opposed to just spending an hour with her. This was supposed to be a great night out. We ended up going down to the off-licence. I got a bottle of vodka and Margaret got a bottle of whiskey. And between the two of us we went through half the bottles each watching videos on the television. And then it got too late. Margaret didn't want to have sex then. When I touched her she, you know, she got ratty with me. When I went upstairs Margaret was naked in the bed and I got in beside her and when I put my hand on her she said, "Don't do that. If you do that again you'll sleep in the other room." I remember it was the night of the Presidential elections when Mary Robinson was going forward and I had to vote because I wanted to vote for Mary Robinson.'

On another morning, after a sexually more eventful night, the pair got into Margaret's car and went to the nearby Nutgrove Shopping Centre *en route* to the city centre and a shift at the Kasbah. It was prove a turning point in the life of Margaret 'Poppy' Healy although she didn't know it at the time. Said Keegan, 'She drove to the Social Welfare offices at the Nutgrove. It was a Wednesday and I knew already that Wednesday was women's day for picking up the dole. I never knew that she was on the dole but I noticed that she didn't make any purchases when she came out of Welfare and went into the shopping centre. And, eh, a lot of things clicked in my mind and I was able to remember much later the sequence of events there – that she had gone in and hadn't bought anything so I assumed that she was on the dole as well as working. She used to make a good £500 a week. Easily. Possibly more but it was a minimum of £500 because she was doing three men a day. That would be about £90 a day.' Early into the New Year these thoughts were committed to print in the form of a letter to the Revenue Commissioners and the seeds of the destruction of the Kasbah were sown.

The bringing of a client home is strictly taboo for the girls in the vice trade. Said Pia Masterson, 'It's just one thing you never, ever do, you never let them know where you live.' Linda Lavelle took some risks in this respect, but never with a character as manifestly unstable as John Keegan. 'Some men [clients] would know where I live. They are men I have known for years and totally, totally trust. But you must trust them in an area of your life that really they shouldn't know about and that concerns your family.' During the summer of 1991, Linda's partner, Liam, suffered a heart attack. His extended convalescence required her to stay out of the Kasbah for weeks on end. Their youngest child, Greta (not her real name), was then aged three and already showing the same willpower and determination that had kept her mother in fine kilter for all these years. Liam's recuperation was undoubtedly helped by this little gem. But having to mind her in his condition was out of the question. Linda relied on the telephone to ensure the smooth running of her vice dens in both Mountjoy Square and Laura's Studio in Belvedere Place.

Margaret Healy and her lover Little John had effectively taken over as joint managers of both the Kasbah and Laura's. 'That's how it all started, that's how the rot set in,' said Linda Lavelle 'Poppy and Little John had become too dangerous because they knew too much, they knew everything: about the clients, about the other girls, about what really goes on, especially in the Kasbah. They knew everything. They had the evidence to hang us all and they hung us all in one way or another. I had warned Poppy about Little John. I had bad feelings about him. I thought he must be robbing all the money he was throwing around and that there was going to be some retaliation about it sooner or later. She assured me that he would be shown the door as soon as his money ran out.'

Margaret Healy was true to her word. As his £12,000 employment settlement figure inexorably marched its way to zero, Poppy's affections for her 'honey' Little John began to diminish commensurately. Despite his paranoia, his clinical anxiety and schizophrenia, John Keegan was and is a highly intelligent and articulate man. It didn't take him long to see that, as far as he and Poppy were concerned, the end was nigh (although he steadfastly believes to this day that their relationship was sustained – on her part as well as his – by more than something as crass as the thickness of his wallet.)

> She used to kiss and call me honey
> But that was when I still had money
> My vice girl from Rathfarnham
> After a year she wasn't quite so nice
> And all her love had turned to ice
> She put a knife into my heart
> And from her lips I had to part

> *My vice girl from Rathfarnham*
> *Soon Miss Poppy had to leave the Square*
> *And many blonde ladies had to change their hair*
> *Some had to pay a really small fine*
> *But the Queen of Hearts still walks the line*
> *Without Miss Poppy from Rathfarnham*

John Keegan's angst at being slowly and, to him at least, unjustly prised out of Margaret Healy's life led to a prolific spate of letter and poem writing. The poem above, entitled *Poppy Cock*, was sent to the home of Linda Lavelle, 'the Queen of Hearts'. There were other odes as time went on and the financial well became drier and drier, some of them more menacing and less reflective, such as the one to Teasy, who was, in fact, also Linda Lavelle.

> *Clever Teasy from the Border*
> *Some tender love is in order*
> *Please don't put me on cold ice*
> *Dressed to kill you look so nice*
> *Really need your woman's love*
> *Coming at me from above*
> *Swinging right before [my] eyes*
> *High above those golden thighs*
> *I am yours to command*
> *And for you I always stand*
> *Give me milk its what I need*
> *And I will give you demon seed*
> *Clever Teasy from the Border*
> *I can carry out your order*
> *Let me taste your Golden Melons*
> *I can save you from these felons*

By November of 1990 Little John had less than £1,500 of his Post Office pay-off left. The rift between himself and Poppy

Healy was noticeable, not only to Linda but to the other women at the Kasbah as well. He was desperate – desperate at the looming prospect of being left alone again. On one level he knew that Poppy was likely to be gone as soon as the money ran out: that was the deal and he often talked to Linda about it in client terms assuring her that there wouldn't be any problems regarding the relationship he was having with the manageress of the Kasbah, as both he and Poppy saw her, when the money ran out. Linda Lavelle did not believe him. More worrying, she did not know what to believe: she had no idea which way Poppy and, more especially, Little John, would jump as soon as that day – the day the money finally ran out – arrived.

She was to find out soon enough.

Little John Keegan's visit to the Kasbah shortly after lunch time on Christmas Eve 1990, marked the final act in his pathetic and potentially explosive liaison with Margaret Healy. Linda Lavelle let him in but once Poppy clapped eyes on her suitor, she turned to Linda with the dread ultimatum that she would leave the Kasbah for good within ten minutes unless Keegan took himself off immediately. She didn't address her former lover at all: there was no eye contact. Linda just looked at the two of them. John Keegan turned and left without saying a word, heading straight for his old watering hole, the Waldorf on the quays.

One of the barmaids in the hotel had got to know him reasonably well over the years. It was primarily because of this fact, and, of course because it was the season to be merry, that she didn't refuse him yet another large bottle of Guinness as he sat slumped in a corner making too much noise, even for a Christmas Eve in a boozer in Dublin. She could not make sense of his angry rantings; about what he was going to do to the Square, to Margaret Healy and to the Kasbah. And he was laughed at by passing Yuletide tipplers when he sought to tell them his tale of woe about being barred from a brothel by his girlfriend on Christmas Eve.

A few days into the New Year he had more messages for Linda Lavelle, only this time Little John Keegan was sober and at his most destructive. He told her that he was going to report Poppy to the police and to the Social Welfare. He was bitter and angry and brimming with self-justification. Linda Lavelle chided him for threatening to kiss-and-tell but not before she listened to him for hours about that 'rotten bitch' Poppy who was running out on him. Her worst fears, she thought as she sat there patiently without saying a word in the weird surroundings of his bedroom while his unsuspecting mother pottered around downstairs, were beginning to unfold. He was particularly hurt and angered by the scene in the Kasbah on Christmas Eve, he said, when Poppy threatened to leave the minute she set eyes on him. 'I never loved her,' he told Linda, 'but I had some genuine warm feelings for her. Sometimes I think Poppy never even liked me, even before the relationship started to show visible cracks. I was happy just to be around her; to get some warm feeling. Why had she to go and treat me like someone who had just gone through her handbag?'

The notion of involving the police first occurred to John Keegan on that Christmas Eve, 1990. Before going official, he decided to use the option as a bargaining ploy with Linda Lavelle: in return for his silence, certain conditions must be met. It almost worked. Using all her diplomatic skills, Linda had extracted his undertaking that there would be no information or complaints passed to the Social Welfare, the police, or anyone else for that matter. In return, she guaranteed that Poppy Healy would behave well towards him (whatever that was supposed to mean). 'No great favours,' John Keegan said, reiterating the terms, 'just that she treats me with respect.' Poppy wasn't even aware that a deal had been struck until later when Linda pointed out to her the potential for disaster that was within his ken for everyone who had anything to do

with the Kasbah. Inevitably, the pact came unstuck in a matter of weeks. Poppy had tried to act more civilly in his
company but she was either unable or unwilling – or both – to
keep the pretence going for very long. 'I didn't expect her to do
the business with me. I didn't expect any great favours. I just
wanted a bit of friendliness from her but she became as frosty
as ever after a while,' John Keegan said later.

His remarks showed a profound naivety as to the dynamics
of prostitution as I had come to understand them. Traits such
as friendliness, loyalty and goodwill, are virtually never shown
towards clients in the worlds of the Poppy Healys and others
in hired vice. That is not a criticism, just a fact due more to
the lifestyles than the personalities of women in prostitution.
For them, it can't, I believe, be any other way if they are to survive. This phenomenon was first revealed to me at a very early
stage in the processes of this book when Linda spoke to me
about how good the girls in the business had been to her
through her days of strain and sorrow as the trial of Marion
Murphy unfolded in the dock of Court Number 13 in the
Central Criminal Court. She was referring to five ladies who
sat in the recesses of the public gallery during the three-day
trial. 'They were great skins. They were there when they were
needed.' She had, in fact, paid them each £100 a day for their
attendance in court – a figure that did not include taxis to and
from the court and the supply of hats and sunglasses to protect
their identities from prying photographers, astute policemen
and even more astute acolytes of the Legion of Mary complete
with their mantras of conversion from sin. And she saw no
conflict in acknowledging what she saw as uncompromised
loyalty from her fellow prostitutes with the fact that she had
paid them quite handsomely for their attendance. 'Sure I'd
have to pay them, for God's sake. They would have been out
of pocket. And, anyway, I wouldn't have any of them be able
to say that they turned up in support of me and I didn't give
them a penny. I won't have them saying that.'

(At least these loyal women fared better than the taxi man who brought one of the women home from court and was spotted doing so on television news that night by his wife. The couple, whose relationship was already strained, split up shortly after the incident with her accusing him of keeping wicked company. The episode distressed the prostitutes. Said Pia Masterson, 'the poor fucker got the marching cards from his wife because she must have thought he was in cahoots with us, that he was a client of ours. The poor man, I really feel sorry for him. We'd never seen him before in our lives. He was never a client of any of the massage parlours.')

On the morning of 28 February 1991, John Keegan left his home, a small working-class residential pocket in Clontarf just off the seafront and two miles north of the city centre to post two more letters penned in his disturbingly erotic bedroom the night before. But this time they weren't poetic entreaties to Linda Lavelle. With Poppy's position now clearly stated, things had gone too far. The letters were made out to the Revenue Commissioners and to the police. They simply stated that Margaret Healy was a prostitute and worked with other prostitutes at a massage parlour in Mountjoy Square West, which was really a brothel known as the Kasbah. The letter to the police was made in the form of an official complaint: the importance of this is significant in that it meant the police had to act if they believed it to be a bona fide complaint. John Keegan was at his most dangerous on those occasions when he managed to subsume his retching emotional self-doubt and replace it with the fires of bitterness and anger.

Linda Lavelle was still trying to renegotiate terms for her disaffected and potentially dangerous client at this time and Little John was beginning to enjoy her increasing sense of desperation. In one of his many soured monologues, he claimed that Poppy had overcharged him. How he could rationalise this no one knows. Linda said that she could arrange to make up for this matter in some way, presumably by providing girls for sex on an amiable settlement-in-kind basis. She was desperately worried that Keegan was about to blow the whistle on ten of her best years. She was not aware that the Armageddon on her empire of vice was already set in motion. Little John basked in the attention and power he commanded again, although by now he was penniless having been cut off the dole, and refused on principle to collect Social Welfare payments. He enjoyed pulling the strings. 'Did Poppy always have false teeth?' he asked Linda sarcastically. Of her offers of proposed arrangements for him with other girls, he said, 'I would have preferred to have Poppy [back] than have a free roll in the hay for a few days or weeks.' He even went as far as to question whether Linda used drugs while on duty in the Kasbah. (It was well known to everyone that Linda Lavelle's only vice was vice. She is a non-smoker and virtual teetotaller.)

Margaret Healy received something of a shock when she arrived at the welfare centre in Rathfarnham on 3 March 1991, to find that her payments had been stopped: the instant she had put him out of the Kasbah for good Little John Keegan had lost any emotional or romantic interest in her; he was now in a position to cause real problems and he struck first, naturally enough, at his former paid paramour.

Three days later the police raided the Kasbah.

Little John Keegan spoke to Poppy Healy for the last time on Holy Thursday in March of 1991 in a telephone call to the Kasbah. He wrote to Linda Lavelle afterwards. 'She [Poppy] did not seem repentant or contrite at all. I decided not to tell her what plans I had in store. You know me, Linda, after a few beers I can't contain myself. She said that if I was with other girls [prostitutes] not to mention her or discuss her. I was, of course, thinking to myself, you can rely on me, Poppy, to put it out on the BBC. Would you have paid me any more attention if I had warned you that Poppy could cost you the business because she couldn't treat people half decently?' John Keegan concluded that letter which was written on 19 November 1991, 'The way she'd treated me you'd think I had asked her for free bed and board and all the extras. It would've made my day if the story had a happy ending and Poppy had been a good fairy instead of the wicked witch. Goodbye, Linda, XXX.'

If 1992 was the *annus horribilis* for the Queen of England, then the previous year was the *annus horribilis* for the queen of vice in Ireland, Linda Lavelle. The police raid on the basement of 60B Mountjoy Square West in March was a fairly tame affair. Names and addresses were taken. Margaret Healy was brought down to Fitzgibbon Street police station where she made a full confession. On 13 May of that year she was fined £80 after pleading guilty in the lower courts to keeping a brothel, to wit the Kasbah. Her defending solicitor, Jim Orange, said that Ms Healy was a former book keeper. He told the court, 'this is clearly a descent from grace.'

By this time Little John was in clear collusion with the police. He started describing himself to Linda in his letters and telephone calls as The Inch-High Private Eye and cautioning her about the insecurity of using '088' mobile phone systems. But it was less a case of friendly counsel than of vindictive taunting as one of his letters reveals. 'You really must be careful with these mobile phones, [you] never know who is around the corner with a personal stereo! Maybe I should ask [Detective Kevin] Fields to return my old radio, even if it was only Hong Kong rubbish.'

The fruits of John Keegan's campaign to wreak havoc on the massage parlours of Dublin bore fruit at precisely 2pm on the afternoon of Wednesday, 4 September 1991. Ironically, it was his former 'lover' Poppy Healy who secured access for Detective Inspector Michael Duggan, a student police officer called Angela Willis and Detective James J. Barry, the assigned Exhibits Officer. They arrived via the raid on Laura's Studio

Ladies of the Kasbah

where both Linda and Poppy had been involved. Poppy told them she would get access for them to the Kasbah; Marion Murphy was there, too, and her offer to accompany the police to 60B was turned down after she had warned the girls through a window in Belvedere Place that a police raid was taking place. Youthful officer Willis hadn't long to wait before knowing for sure she was in the right place. A cassette folder bearing the words, 'Huge Bras Number 4' on a bedside locker in a corner of the large front room was handed over to the Exhibits Officer, as was a copy of *The Business Man's Guide*, magazine advertisements for 'The Kasbah Massage Parlour' along with sundry items such as baby oil, talcum powder, and a large quantity of towels. Two prostitutes who were in the premises at the time, Patricia (not her real name) and Liz Brophy, agreed to accompany the police to Fitzgibbon Street police station in Liz's beloved but ageing silver Ford Escort where they made statements confirming their vocations in vice, although Patricia denied that she had ever offered full sex to clients.

Liz, a stunningly attractive woman who had earned the name of Ice Cold Madam because of her detachment from and, some would say cynicism for both her fellow prostitutes and the clients, would later take the witness stand against Marion Murphy in the Kasbah trial. She arrived at the Kasbah on 20 March 1990, after working as a prostitute in brothels in Baggot Lane and South William Street owned by County Clare born vice baron Tom McDonnell. One of McDonnell's muscular consultants hit her on the side of the head with a wooden plank after she had refused to have sex with him. Naturally enough, she felt it was time to consider different employment prospects. While in the Kasbah, Liz – she also used the names Jill, Sharon, Kim, or Hayley – provided a full range of sexual services to male clients.

Patricia arrived at the Kasbah after living in Dublin for a year and a half. She had a 17-month-old baby and was on the dole until the day she answered a coded advertisement in *In Dublin* magazine and started work at the Kasbah in July 1991. She came to live in Dublin from her County Tipperary home in February 1990, around the same time that she had given birth to a son. She had just turned twenty years of age.

Police video surveillance had been placed on the Kasbah at the direction of Detective Inspector Michael Duggan on Friday 5 July 1991, and commenced at precisely 4.15pm. Under the supervision of Detective Sergeant Timothy Daly, officers Gus Keane and Kevin Fields began the covert video monitoring from the back of an unmarked white Hi-Ace van parked sixty feet from the premises at 60B Mountjoy Square West. On that first date alone, officers Fields and Keane observed five males entering and leaving the basement of 60B between 4.15pm and 7.46pm. As well as logging the information through the lens of a video camera, Detective Fields took copious notes on the clients: their features; what they were wearing and, of course, the make and registration number of their vehicles.

The police claim that a similar operation was mounted much later at Laura's Studio in Belvedere Place, which also included the use of video surveillance equipment, has never been confirmed, although it is known that an operation involving the logging of clients' movements to and from that premises was part of the overall operation mounted against Marion Murphy.

In all, a total of 123 men were logged entering and leaving the Kasbah and Laura's Studio between 4.15pm on 5 July 1991 and 3.45pm on 20 August when one stage of the stake-out concluded with the observation of a client who chained his bicycle to the railings outside Belvedere Place and emerged exactly thirty minutes later when he was invited to accompany Messrs Keane and Fields to Fitzgibbon Street as he pushed the unlocked security chain into his coat pocket.

The surveillance operation was centred almost exclusively

on the Kasbah. The number of men observed entering and leaving the premises during the stake-out represented only a tiny fraction of those who actually visited both brothels during that two-and-a-half month period from 5 July to 25 September in which the women of the bordellos conservatively estimate that over 1,500 men had used either or both of the establishments for some form of paid sexual service. The police surveillance exercise rarely lasted more than three hours on any given day and was by no means a seven-day-a-week project.

Margaret Healy's decision to plead guilty and get away with a caution and fine to the charges brought against her was, at the time, par for the course among vice girls in Dublin who were charged with such offences. To contest the charge she would have had the effect of opening up a completely different vista involving a jury, witnesses (in this context a euphemism for clients) and very considerable legal costs with no guarantee of a more favourable court verdict.

By this time the police heat was on the Kasbah like never before in its ten years of free-thinking dreadfulness. Like all good madams, Linda Lavelle had her sources within the police force and outside it who kept her informed of what was going on. (Most of them seemed to be motivated out of a progressive social sense, although one source expected – and received – a more tangible reward for his information by being discreetly and expertly masturbated by the girls in public houses.)

Linda's contacts left her in no doubt that the court case involving Margaret Healy and the Kasbah was only the start of her troubles. In this she blames Margaret Healy and John Keegan in equal measure.

'Poppy gave them [the police] everything. I gave them nothing,' she said referring to Marion Murphy's decision to contest the charges which were levelled against her on 28 January, 1992. 'Poppy colluded with the police. Everything they wanted to know about the girls and the clients came from her and from Little John.' She is in all probability correct. Her excoriation of Margaret Healy has left the Cork woman a *persona non grata* within the world of Dublin prostitution. But blaming her for what she did is not entirely even-handed. Poppy held to her word that Little John would be gone as soon as his money ran out. She was handed to the police by Little John: that she didn't contest the brothel-keeping charges brought against her in relation to the Kasbah had less to do with perceived dishonour by her fellow prostitutes than with personal survival. It was the route taken by virtually all prostitutes faced with the weight of the law bearing down on them. Poppy Healy just didn't have the calibre, the strength and, of course, the finances – to take on the establishment in the way her then landlady, Marion Murphy, did. No one, including Linda Lavelle, really expected Poppy to take any course with the system other than the one she did.

If there is cause to find fault in Margaret Healy in this world of faults, of moving rights and moving wrongs, it is found in her gratuitous petty-mindedness and love of trouble-making, especially with other prostitutes' clients.

It didn't help her case, either, that she took the witness stand in The Kasbah case in 1993. That action was never seen as simply a case of welshing on Linda Lavelle and Marion Murphy. It was perceived by prostitutes in massage parlours throughout the country as someone pulling the plug on a way of life that was infinitely more acceptable than working the streets. And experience has shown that perception to be well founded.

What was utterly remarkable and inexplicable to many, particularly those outside the orbit of the Kasbah, was Linda Lavelle's relationship with the treacherous Little John Keegan during and after the trial. One would have expected him to be about as popular and as safe as a bunny rabbit among Rottweilers. To some degree this was true: many prostitutes once attached to the Kasbah still have difficulty in getting his

name out and staying seated at the same time. Yet his relationship with Linda and a few of the other girls continued
during these worst of times. He maintained his prolific letter-
writing to her, his apologies laced with barbs and sexual
innuendo directed at both her and Poppy Healy. Linda
responded by meeting him several times at his home in
Clontarf. She even gave him money and cigarettes. Once she
took him out for a meal when his dole payments were
suddenly cut off and he refused on principle to accept inter-
regnum State payments.

For hours she would listen patiently to his self-pitying talk,
which included blaming his mother for what he saw as her role
in bringing about his pathetic state. He complained of his
problems relating to members of the opposite sex; his abject
remorse for getting Linda into the trouble she was currently
facing at the hands of the Irish police force; and, of course, he
talked about his continuing fascination for a woman called
Margaret Healy.

By March of 1992 the small bedroom of John Keegan's terraced home in Clontarf was saturated with paraphernalia of
twisted sexual fantasy. Murals with a strong Nazi leitmotif of
blonde women covered the four walls. His mother's expres-
sions of disapproval were met by the sarcastic and anger-filled
response that he could always repaint his ladies naked with
their internal organs sketched in from medical text books if
she complained too much. Little John even constructed a life-
sized doll of Poppy, complete with breasts and other female
appendages. ('She never gets a headache,' he once told Linda.)
The doll was meant to complement a picture he had drawn of
Poppy – half cartoon, half 'modern art' – wrapped only in a
towel with one of her breasts exposed.

It was within the strangeness, the madness, of these four
walls that Linda sat for hours listening to John Keegan's tale of
wretchedness. He would assure her that the cops could never
call him as a witness against her, no matter what he had told

them. 'They'd really get a dressing down for that when it came out that I had a psychiatric history.' He reassured her that he was taking legal advice about the possibility of withdrawing any statements to the police that he had made against her and the Kasbah's landlady, Marion Murphy. He even said that if he was called to give evidence against her he would refuse point-blank to open his mouth, risking jail for contempt of court. The only thing that mattered to him was, he said, Linda Lavelle's forgiveness.

'You know, Linda, I couldn't live with myself if I destroy you the way they want me to. I'm sorry enough already, even if I can't express it. Will you still talk to me when it's all over, Linda?'

In a move hardly designed to make her feel more comforted and supported by his new contriteness, Little John said that he would do whatever he could and if it wasn't enough, 'I'll be looking for a rope.' As always, Linda just listened, interjecting quietly sometimes to impress upon Little John the dire position he had placed her in by ratting to the police about Poppy and by extension, herself, Marion Murphy and the Kasbah. Yes, yes, he was aware of all that, he said. He was truly sorry. He would love to take it all back . . . but he would still 'find a rope' if she didn't continue to talk to him.

> You raise me up – I brought you down
> A fallen angel with golden crown
> And with you I cannot live
> Unless my sin you can forgive

What Linda Lavelle's motives were in keeping contact with and acting as a benefactor to John Keegan after all he had done to this point are quite inexplicable. Part of it was obviously an exercise in survival as she sifted through the wreckage of his terrible deeds of betrayal to see what, if anything, could be redeemed from the situation in time for the court case involving Marion Murphy. But even at that early stage it was by and large a lost cause trying to get him somehow to ameliorate the situation. Police sources had made it clear that Little John Keegan was no longer all that important and that 'the big guns' in the police force and the Department of Justice were by that stage calling the shots and they intended moving in on the Kasbah. Little John had become surplus to police evidence-gathering requirements the day the video cameras started rolling in Mountjoy Square

And long after it was all over and the Kasbah was nothing but a memory of some other time in her life, Linda Lavelle was still befriending Little John Keegan, 'That dotty little brothel crawler who closed down seven massage parlours in the space of a fortnight,' she had once said in a fit of pique. Keegan remembers her magnanimity this way, 'Linda was very good to me. I mean she used to bring me out, even after the Kasbah was closed and the trial process was still pending. Once she brought me out to the Clarence Hotel and we had lunch there and a bottle of wine as well. Other times she brought me out to McDonalds. I remember once she took me to Malahide [a seaside town north of Dublin city] with her daughter, Greta. Greta went swimming and then afterwards we went up to McDonalds in Artane and she bought me burgers and chips. And, ha, I was wearing a German army shirt at the time and Greta said to me, "Are you a guard? – me mammy [*sic*] hates guards!" Linda brought me other places, too . . . she can be a very generous woman. She brought me out to coffee shops all over Dublin and we'd just have coffee and cigarettes. And she'd always make sure I'd had cigarettes because at the time I had no money. I was completely broke. She was very generous but she was a very determined woman and at the same time she can be ruthless. You know. Ruthless.'

A few weeks after the court case had ended Linda Lavelle brought me out to Keegan's home with a view my writing a story on the grotesque Nazi paintings and the Poppy doll. We had met earlier that day in Linda's premises in Belvedere Place along with Vikki O'Toole and Pia Masterson. The three women were very clear about their motives then: they wanted this D.L.B.C. embarrassed and held to public ridicule and it wasn't difficult to see the origins of their sense of revenge. For twenty minutes or so we sat in the large room in Belvedere Place. Little John was there, having previously agreed with Linda to allow me to do the story. He was smoking the girls' cigarettes and speaking about wanting to do the interview in order to profess in public his sorrow for shopping Linda, to the police and, in a sense, to the Irish public. The girls all sat around nodding their heads in recognition at his noble intent before Vikki said, 'Right, let's get in the fucking cars and fucking go.' She couldn't wait to see the tables turned and she told me later that she'd heard 'Too many of his fucking "I'm so sorry" holier than thou fucking speeches.'

Nor could Linda Lavelle ever explain her ambivalence towards Little John Keegan. I wondered at the time whether it had something to do with the one character trait they had in common and which marked them out from the vast majority of people: that they were on the outside of life as the rest of us know it and they were looking in. Linda once said of her Discipline clients, 'I get a buzz from all of them because they all act differently.' She is inexorably drawn to the clients she calls 'the loopers' and 'the nutters', the men – and women – who behave outside recognised and accepted patterns. Although only into straight sex, Little John was one such soul.

For a journalist covering the Kasbah trial and the incidents which led up to it, the Little John story was of considerable significance. The public had just witnessed a three-day court case involving massive expense. Questions were being asked as to why such an operation was necessary at all. The police refused to talk off the record or on the record about the dynamics behind the court case. In over twenty years in journalism I have never encountered such a complete lack of cooperation from the police than on the story of the Kasbah. The resistance was encapsulated for me by one of the detectives at the centre of the investigation, Gus Keane, who told me, 'You have all [the information] you need from the trial. There's nothing else to it. I won't be talking any further about it than that.' The detective was just doing his job. Much later, Keane's fellow officer, Detective Kevin Fields, explained that he could not assist me and invited me instead to make a formal request for police cooperation through the press office. He, too, was just doing his job. My application to the police press office was not responded to. In such circumstances, John Keegan was the only person who could provide some idea as to what was behind the Kasbah raid, if anything.

Keegan was only referred to once during the three-day trial of Marion Murphy, and then not by name. It came by way of a reponse from Detective Kevin Fields when Judge Buchanan noted what he called the 'enormous amount of police time and public money' that had gone into the investigation. Detective Fields sad that the operation was initiated following a series of written complaints by a dissatisfied client of the Kasbah Health Studio who was mentally unbalanced and who had also sent a series of letters to the Minister for Justice and the Garda Commissioner.

Suggestions that John Keegan had reported Margaret Healy and the Kasbah to the Department of Justice, the Garda Commissioner, the Department of Social Welfare and the Revenue Commissioners flattered the ex Post Office worker's efforts at thoroughness. Initially, only two letters were sent out, one to the police at Fitzgibbon Street Station and the other to the Revenue Commissioners. Only the letter to the tax authorities was actually signed by Keegan, the other was an anonymous albeit highly detailed and skilful piece of writing.

Linda Lavelle is blunt in her anger at the legal process. 'There must be hundreds of people writing daily to Ray Burke [the then Minister for Justice] and the police authorities with genuine situations, genuine problems, genuine emergencies and complaints. Then they get this unsigned letter from a dotty little brothel crawler and they send in the fucking police to close down a massage parlour that Fields himself said in court wasn't bothering anyone. [What he actually said was that the Kasbah had been a low-key operation before the written complaints and did not seem to be bothering anyone.] Where the fuck is the justice in that?' She added, 'And when the matter comes to the courts the girls and the Madams are the ones that are named. We're the ones who suffer the indignity of having our names and addresses and pictures splashed all over the newspapers while the clients of the place get the benefit of an arrangement between the defence solicitors, the State's solicitors and the judge which sees to it that they are not identified. Remember, it takes two to fucking tango: those men came to us for something; we didn't go to them.

'Why the hell are they getting that sort of treatment?

'And why the hell are the women in this business all left toeing the line for the men? Always?'

Chapter Eighteen

Truth And Treason

The brothel shift outside the Kasbah on Tuesday, 20 August 1991, started no differently than other such posting in Mountjoy Square for Detectives Keane, Fields and student officer Angela Willis. They observed three men entering and leaving the Kasbah between 5.10pm and 8pm. Shortly after 7pm, Detective Keane and student officer Willis approached one of the men they had seen leaving the basement brothel and heading in the direction of offices in Belvedere Place. Detective Keane produced identification and invited the man to make a statement in Fitzgibbon Street police station which he agreed to do. He was to join the ranks of thirteen men who agreed to give such statements which later took the form of depositions to the lower courts and part of the Book of Evidence against Marion Murphy.

What neither Keane nor Willis could have realised at the time was that the man, a high-powered official in the Dublin power structures of the GAA, was a student of the most depraved and objectionable form of masochistic sex as a client of Linda Lavelle and her girls at the Kasbah.

His deposition to the lower courts and his statement to the police on the night of Tuesday, 20 August 1991 which was given as police surveillance of the brothels continued, gave no indication that he was anything other than a client of a massage parlour who indulged in straightforward sexual acts. Nothing could be further from the truth, according to his women servers. It is due to the persona of this man, and many others like him – scions of the respectable, acceptable, establishment – that the seeds of anger and resentment at the treatment of Linda Lavelle and other prostitutes are found. It is this perception that somehow the girls are immoral – sluts – while their male clients have temporarily veered off the moral pathway, that is perhaps the greatest injustice committed against the prostitutes.

Keegan made his apology to Linda and the rest of the vice women publicly as promised in an interview I conducted with him shortly after the trial. He consented to be photographed in his very strange bedroom with the Nazi murals, most of which resembled Margaret Healy, painted on every available square inch of space. He posed with his Poppy doll. He joked again about her never having headaches. He walked me out to my car and bade farewell. As he did so Linda walked over to him and asked him whether he would like to join her and the girls for a few drinks – on them, of course – I refused a similar invitation on the grounds that I had to get back to the office and write up the story. At first Little John seemed reluctant until Vikki, of all people, used some mothering charm to persuade him to join them. It was another poignant example of the great paradox of these prostitute women's humanity, motivated simultaneously by revenge and genuine concern for another human whom Linda and Vikki and some of the other women of the Kasbah saw as lamentable and in need of their support.

One of the girls, Pia, whom I asked about this later, knowingly joked, 'We're carers of men, Dave, with all their problems and situations. Little John is a proper bastard, make no mistake. But he didn't pretend to be something he wasn't.'

Pia had touched upon an issue seen by Linda Lavelle and the prostitutes close to her as one of the great acts of treason in the whole affair: that of the depositions by the thirteen clients who confirmed to the police and to the District Court in their Statements of Evidence that they had visited either Laura's Studio or the Kasbah in Mountjoy Square West.

'They're bastards, all of them,' said Linda. 'They didn't tell it like it was for them, what was really going on. They told the police that they had straight sex and masturbation and that. It wasn't like that at all. They gave the impression that the women were in it just for the money and that left a totally false impression. Most of these bastards were in the Kasbah because they were perverts. It gives the impression that we were the wrong-doers and they were just poor men looking for a bit on the side – a bit of straight sex. The country should know about these perverts, the country should know that they are perverts and that they came to us looking to satisfy their perversions.'

I wasn't sure what point Linda was trying to make. Surely she could not expect her clients, those whom she and the other women claimed were Slaves, masochists, and sundry perverts, to pour their hearts out to the police in written statements? I became less confused when I reminded myself as I had to time and time again while in the company of the Kasbah women that logic had little or no control over their lives; that it was never about Linda or anyone else expecting someone to act in a certain way. No, it was about something much bigger than that. It was about how society perceives them, it was about what they so strongly believe is an injustice in society's attitude that is perpetrated against all prostitutes.

This statement given by a client – A.M.C. – to the police at Fitzgibbon Street station, is typical:

On the 1st August 1991 I arrived in Dublin around 12.30pm. I drove to a premises I had seen advertised in the *Golden Pages*. The premises is situated at 60 Mountjoy Square. It was advertised as a Massage and Sauna. I parked my car opposite the premises and put money into the meter for a waiting period of two hours. I went to the premises . . . I rang the bell and the door was opened to me by a young lady in her late twenties. She had a skirt on and a top. She was dressed decently. I was invited in . . . As I entered to the left there was an area . . . curtained off. I think it was light brown. It ran for abut thirteen feet and opened up into a narrow corridor. To the left of this corridor were some small cubicles, I think three. Across on the right was a shower and a toilet. The girl that admitted me didn't give her name. She told me that there was two other girls. She said did I want to see the other girls and I said yes.

They came and I was introduced to them, Jill and Tina. Jill was wearing a towel which covered her with reasonable modesty and [Tina] was dressed normally. I said I'd like to have Jill, the girl with the towel. She was aged about twenty, she might have been eighteen. . . she was pretty with short blonde hair. Jill gave me a quotation. Before this the girl who admitted me gave me a quotation of £15 for a straight massage and also informed me that there was extras. Jill said that in addition to the £15 there was an extra for strip relief, that's the expression she used. She quoted further prices, oral sex for £25 extra, convention[al] sex, I can't remember how much that was, and finally for a mixture of oral and conventional sex, I think she said £40. I opted for what they call strip relief. Prior to Jill quoting me I was instructed as to where the shower is by Jill, so I had a shower in the shower room opposite the cubicles.

When I returned from the shower room I just had a towel around me . . . before I went to the shower I paid over £15 Irish to Jill. I went into the cubicle. The only furniture in the room was a flat bunk, no headboards or pillows, a small portable T.V. . . . The text of the T.V. was explicit scenes of a sexual nature, involving men and women. There was sound but it was very bad quality. I was sitting naked on the couch when Jill returned. I was watching T.V. She had the towel around her when she came in. She locked the door behind her. These cubicles are totally enclosed . . . When she came in I lay on my tummy and faced the T.V. . . . She dropped the towel and sat down on the bed. I saw her naked. She gave me a massage on my back. She used talc, no oil. This lasted a few minutes. After a few minutes she asked me to turn over.

She massaged my tummy and penis using oil this time . . . There was very little conversation between us. She masturbated me until I was erect with this oil. I didn't ejaculate at this stage. She then said would I like oral sex as I hadn't come. She put a condom on my penis. I don't know where she got it from. She then put my penis in her mouth and there was no climax – for the record. She said at one stage, 'We have been going for twenty minutes and I don't think you're going to come,' so it was left at that. She asked me for the extra for oral sex. I gave her £25 and she left the room. I had another shower and dressed and left. I saw Jill on the way out and she was still wearing her towel. She said, 'I hope to see you again.' I told her how much prettier she looked in the daylight and I left. Then I saw you [the policeman] approaching me . . .

The Irish penchant for both creativity and haggling over the price didn't desert another visitor to the Kasbah – Mr M.T. from Galway – who confessed to the police abut an episode in Dublin in early summer, 1991:

I rang the bell and was admitted by a young girl I now know as Kim. She gave me a full massage, she then turned me over and caught a hold of my penis. She was rubbing it and pulling it, she was rubbing oil into my testicles and I got a horn [erection]. She then offered me full sex. She said it was a fiver for a hand job which is a wank, a tenner for a blow job and £30 for full sex. I made a bargain with her and she gave me full sex for £20. The procedure is you walk in the door, she shows you a room, she looks for her £15 for a massage, you give her this, then she leaves the room and says if you want a shower you can have one and lie up on the bed.

When she came back I was lying up on the bed with my underwear on and she came in and started to massage me, she offered me oil or powder. I chose oil, after a few minutes of massaging my back, my chest, then she asked if I wanted my underwear taken off. All during this there was a blue movie on in the corner, there was a big black fellow riding the backside off a young one. Anyway, she took my underwear off, after I'd agreed a price of £20 for a bit of everything . . . That was three months ago.

Now, on 5th/8/91 I called again to 60 Mountjoy Square and asked for Kim. An older woman had answered the door. She had blonde hair, glasses and was plain looking. Then Kim came out and brought me to a cubicle with a blue movie on in it. It was dark and seedy with red and white lights on. I had full sex again with a blow job and oil and the works . . . The whole session cost me £35 . . . I would describe Kim as 20 years approximately, with short blonde hair, good looking, with [a] nice body. I think she has a Tipperary accent. When I left today I walked around to Gardiner Place to where my car was parked . . .

A well known medical figure – A.M. – was another who made a statement to the police about his visit to the Kasbah on 13 August 1991.

Prior to my going I knew that I could have a variety of sexual reliefs, hand relief, oral relief or full sex. I became aware of 60B from the *Golden Pages*. In any event, I parked my motorcycle and went downstairs, rang the bell. The door was opened to me by a girl with dyed blonde hair, about ten-and-a-half stone, around 5'10", in her early twenties, with a short skirt and top. There was a curtain on the left as you go in. Through a chink in the curtain I could see a man and a woman. I was led to a cubicle, the first of three on my left. It had a low bed, an armchair and pale yellow light. I waited in the cubicle about three minutes. Then the same girl came back. I asked for a massage. She said we're not qualified massage therapists, [and that] most men come here for the extras. I inquired about the extras. I was told £15 for hand relief, £20 for oral relief, and £30 for full sex. I opted for hand relief. I gave her £30 on request and she told me to undress. She came back. I lay face down and she caressed me without oil or talc. She undressed after she came in, I saw her naked. I turned over on my back and she went straight to work to masturbation. She put no condom on me. I climaxed about five minutes after she began masturbating me . . . I left and as I approached the door I noticed the curtain pulled back. The girl who gave me hand relief was again dressed. She was sitting beside two other women on a sofa.

Perhaps Pia Masterson wasn't really joking after all when she laughed about being carers. Perhaps she and the other prostitutes felt that their 'caring' had been violated by the content of the Statements of Evidence, all of which implied straightforward sexual encounters.

On the other hand, Little John's betrayal was something that could be condoned by the prostitutes because he was always on the outside, just like Linda, just like Pia, just like them, 'underdogs', as Linda Lavelle once said.

The GAA figure and the rest of the witnesses had lost their franchise to sin against the sinners.

For they pretended they had hardly sinned at all.